SELF-MADE
Wellionaire™

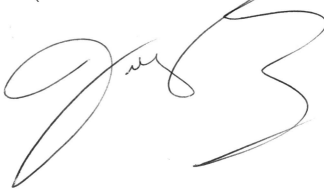

To Melissa,
Wishing you
all the wellth
in the world ☺

Cover design by Jane Ashley
Interior design by Sheryl Kober
Illustrations by Rob Lang
Photos by Lisi Wolf

To contact the publisher, visit
FLOWEROFLIFEPRESS.COM

To contact the author, visit
JILLGINSBERG.COM

Library of Congress Control Number: 2016938885
Flower of Life Press, Lyme, CT.

ISBN-13: 978-0692689455
ISBN-10: 0692689451

Printed in the United States of America

SELF-MADE
Wellionaire™

Get off Your Ass(et),
Reclaim Your Health,
and Feel Like a
Million Bucks

Jill Ginsberg

FLOWER OF LIFE
PRESS.

Voices of Transformation

Praise for *Self-Made Wellionaire*

Inspiring, motivating and wildly funny, *Self-Made Wellionaire* is the wellness book you've been searching for. Jill Ginsberg will not only help you create a better life but a better mind to go with it. This book is about the whole picture, not just how to make more money or acheive the perfect bikini bod. When you get your head straight, everything comes together and Jill will give you the tools to get you there. Her wicked humor doesn't hurt, I laughed the whole read!
~Heather K. Terry, founder of NibMor Chocolate and author of
From Broadway to Wall Street

Biz in the front. Party in the back. You're like the freaking mullet of the business world! I'm going to call you Jilly Ray Cyrus.
~someone who spoke to Jill at a bar

I loved this book! As usual, Jill's writing manages to be inspiring, practical and often hilarious. The book is packed with ideas and action steps that are invaluable to anyone interested in ways to live a healthy and happy life.
~Ben Relles, head of Comedy, YouTube

If you want no-nonsense advice from someone who doesn't take crap from anyone (although technically she does pick up a lot of my shit) this is the book for you.
~Jill's dog's subconscious

My wellness account was practically empty; to paraphrase Top Gun, I was writing checks that my body couldn't cash. Luckily Jill Ginsberg has me well on my way to becoming a "Self-Made Wellionaire." The sound strategies and warm humor she offers on every page of her book will land any reader in the wellthiest tax bracket.
~Wendy Shanker, author of *Are You My Guru? How Medicine, Meditation & Madonna Saved My Life*

Jill's book changed my life. Literally. I'm indebted to her. Which is fine because I'm fucking loaded.
~Rich Prosperous, founder of Weeping Zillows

A fun approach to getting healthy, *Self-Made Wellionaire* uses simple business strategies to change how you approach improving your life, with small, actionable steps anyone can achieve.
~Elizabeth Stein, founder + CEO Purely Elizabeth, author of *Eating Purely*

The one book on wellness I'd have if I could have just one. It's the most exciting thing I've read since the 1994 Pennsylvania Drivers Handbook.
~Jill's High School Drivers Ed Teacher

Whether you're the CEO of a company or CEO of your family kitchen, there's something here for you! Jill has taken the best of what she's seen work as an MBA-educated business person and combined it with her nutrition knowledge to deliver simple tips, actions and templates for life success. These practical steps are sprinkled with a healthy dose of humor that will keep you chuckling and engaged on your personal path to Self-made Wellionaire. A brilliant solution for combining the best of both worlds!
~Sue Brown, author of *Simply Sugar Free: Six Simple Steps to Conquer Sugar Addiction*

Jill has done the perfect job of inspiring, teaching, motivating, and guiding those seeking to improve their lives. However, I really wish she wouldn't have used the word "fucking" in Chapter 6.
~Jill's Mom, who doesn't seem to realize that she also just used the word "fucking"

I've read tons of self-help books that don't ever push me to action, but this one is brilliant. Jill is a genius for taking basic business tools and translating them to everyday life to get healthy. And with a nice dose of humor!
~Sarina Godin, president, butter LONDON cosmetics

This book is just the kick in the pants I needed, and it's a fun read. In fact I read the whole thing while I had Jill placed on hold.
~a support technician from Dell

Praise for *Self-Made Wellionaire*

Your body is a factory: It's either running efficiently, and creating more health and vitality for you, or you're running it into the ground—with mismanagement, union strikes, and forced labor. Using time-honored and effective techniques that work in any size business, Jill Ginsberg uses humor and relatable stories to guide you step by step toward creating a healthy lifestyle in any size body. Learn how to run a tight ship (and maybe even get a tight ass in the process) as you discover how to run your body like a boss (the good kind of boss, not the lousy kind). Who knew creating better eating habits and increasing your health currency could actually be both satisfying AND entertaining? Don't just read this book, use it—and you'll soon have a personal health balance sheet that is worthy of a Wellionaire: "rich with energy, health, purpose, and joy"!
~Kris Prochaska, M.A., author of *Life Well Spoken: Free Your Inner Voice and Prosper*

Thanks to *Self-Made Wellionaire*, I'm the lightest and sharpest I've ever been in my adult life.
~a cloud shaped like a porcupine

Buy this book. You'll want to highlight, mark pages, and write your own notes as you create your path to wellness—and the library frowns on that, so you need to own it like Jill's step-by-step advice will have you owning your health. Recommended!
~Anne Weiler, CEO and co-founder, Wellpepper, Inc.

Self-Made Welllionaire provides a humorous roadmap to health that will benefit anyone. Read it yourself and give it to the people you love. Hell, give it to the people you hate, too.
~Harry Bush-Dong, author of *When Good Parents Give Kids Bad Names*

To Orly, Reuben, Jude,
and "The Peach,"
for teaching me the
true definition of wellth

Contents

PART THREE: Live Like a Wellionaire

Foreword

Oftentimes people approach getting healthy and feeling better like a crapshoot.

Not knowing how to "fix" themselves, they may think about making change, but thanks to an overwhelming number of options and a total lack of clarity, they often decide to throw in the towel before ever taking action. This conundrum is hilariously depicted by an article that was published by *The New Yorker* in August 2015 titled *My Brain: The All-Hands Meeting* by Hallie Cantor.

ME: Hey, everyone, thanks for coming. This meeting is just to check in, get updated about what everybody's been working on in the first quarter of the day, and see how we're feeling about the future. Coffee, wanna kick us off?

COFFEE: Sure, thanks. So, my team's been pretty active in Q1. We started out with our regular one cup, and, you know, we weren't seeing immediate results. We're attributing that to a number of factors. Our target is developing a tolerance owing to her unemployment, plus we all know there've been some hiccups in the new sleep schedule.

(Sleep snorts. Coffee pauses.)

COFFEE: —but we're hoping to hit the ground running in Q2 with the second-cup initiative, and build on the foundation that Antidepressants set up.

ANTIDEPRESSANTS: Yeah, thanks, Coffee. Can I get that PowerPoint I e-mailed everyone up on the screen, please? Great. Now, as you can see, our department's not getting the full R.O.I. we once were. Forty milligrams of Cymbalta used to be enough to get her out of bed and to a coffee shop, but increasingly—especially with the overwhelming trend toward mobile—she's just checking her e-mail on her phone and then going back to sleep.

SLEEP: Can I jump in here?

ME: Sure, Sleep, let's hear from you.

SLEEP: Listen, I know my department has been asking for a lot recently. But what do you want me to say? She's unemployed now. That's a new climate for all of us. We've had to adapt. Her sleeping patterns are being completely recalibrated. Seven hours a night isn't gonna fly. We need nine, ten, even eleven hours now.

COFFEE (under its breath): Ridiculous.

SLEEP: And I hate to say it, but, as we enter Q2, the fact is we need a nap.

(Assorted grumbles and groans can be heard around the room.)

SUGAR: We don't need a nap, O.K.? What we need is a pastry.

PROTEIN: Absolutely not. A pastry is a Band-Aid solution! We need scrambled eggs.

ME: Guys, come on. I can't get into this with you two again before lunch. Let's circle back to Coffee's second-cup initiative. Water, how does that look from your end?

WATER: I'm gonna have to strongly advise against it. If the first cup didn't work, why would we double down on that strategy and sink more resources into a second cup? Besides, my team's projections show that more coffee would frankly be counter to our goals at this point.

COFFEE: Excuse me?

WATER: She's tired because she's *dehydrated*. It's always dehydration! How many articles from the Huffington Post's Healthy Living vertical does her mom need to forward her before this sinks in?

COFFEE (sulkily): There's water in coffee, you know.

EXERCISE: I'm with Water. The work my guys are doing is pointless without support in the form of more water! All through Q1, we were busting our ass at yoga class and she couldn't get any of the benefits because she was feeling light-headed from a single Sun Salutation. That's textbook dehydration. I'm sorry, but it is.

SUGAR: Could be low blood sugar.

EXERCISE: It's not.

SUGAR: It could be, though.

WATER: It's not.

ME: All right, let's cool it with the crosstalk, please. I want to go big picture. None of us can deny the negative trends we've been seeing in mood and productivity. Let's do a deep dive. Therapy, what do you have to say?

THERAPY: I know things look stagnant right now, but it's a process. We're pursuing a long-term strategy, and sometimes things have to get worse before they get better. If we just stay the course—

ANTIDEPRESSANTS: Oh, stuff it.

THERAPY: Hey!

ANTIDEPRESSANTS: I'm sick of this asshole taking credit for the work I'm doing! Therapy, have you *ever* gotten concrete results?

THERAPY: I'm dealing with challenges that the rest of you have never had to handle! An off-site partner is not easy to work with, you know. Her Subconscious couldn't even be bothered to dial in to this meeting.

ME: We tried. The connection was bad.

THERAPY: What else is new?

ME: Look, excuses and finger-pointing aren't going to solve anything. Does anyone have any constructive ideas?

(A calm, wise voice speaks up from the back of the room.)

MEDITATION: Pardon me, but may I make a suggestion? If you'd consider bringing me on full time instead of employing me on a sporadic freelance basis, I really think I could help out with some of these issues.

ME: Yeah, yeah. Maybe next quarter.

(Alcohol clears its throat.)

ALCOHOL: I know you already know that we're all dying to contribute more consistently over in my department.

WEED: Ditto.

ME: Thanks, guys. I appreciate that.

WATER: Tell me you're not considering putting those jackasses in charge.

ME: Not in charge. Just . . . maybe they should have a place at the table. Would that be so terrible?

(Suddenly, the door to the conference room bursts open.)

P.M.S.: Sorry, sorry, sorry! Am I late?

ME: Fuck it. Sleep, you're in charge.

Spot on as this piece is, you'll never get clear on what to do or how to do it by just contemplating it. Getting lost in the quagmire of voices living inside the boardroom in your brain, pondering what-if scenarios to the crunch-crunch beat of Pringles won't get you anywhere. Whether you want to feel more energized, lose weight, or learn how to cook something that can't pop out of a toaster, to move forward you have to get out of your head and start taking action.

But you don't have to do it alone. Step by step, this book shows you exactly how to get off your ass(et), reclaim your health and feel like a million bucks.

Introduction

As a kid I didn't get the importance of having a plan.

My version of thinking ahead involved plotting which goodies I could pilfer from my Grandma's purse without getting caught. Like most children, I lived for the moment.

As I got older, I watched many of my peers proceed with confidence, while I flailed around aimlessly waiting for life to direct me. This continued throughout college. I was the person who didn't even have a resume drafted on graduation day (though I did have a plane ticket to Alaska). Forget about actually applying for a job.

Eventually I got tired of waiting for something great to happen. When I was 26, I applied to business school and, two years later, received my MBA from The University of North Carolina at Chapel Hill. There I learned many fundamental skills and a whole new lexicon of obnoxious business clichés, but what stuck with me the most was the importance of having a plan. In the business world, success is carefully managed. It almost never happens accidentally.

After I graduated in 2004, I launched my own food company and sought to sell my salty snacks throughout the land. I had only one goal—to be wealthy. Driven by the almighty dollar, I pimped my tasty wares here, there, and everywhere. Before long, I had an award-winning product line, a plethora of media mentions, including product features in SELF magazine and on "The Rachael Ray Show," and, like any good MBA-hole, a growing ego to show for it. My business was a raging success.

Until it wasn't.

Erratic cash flow, a lack of funding to support growing retail demand, and a full-blown Great Recession sent my company into a downward spiral. Saddled with a ton of debt and thoroughly dethroned, I went to work in Brand Management for a meat snack company. (Never mind that "meat" and "snack" are two words that should never go together.) Less than two years into the job, the flood of fluorescent lighting, a persistent desire to nap under my desk, ten extra pounds, and a chronic longing to see more of my family left me feeling depleted—and desperate to feel better and find something more meaningful than Power-Pointless.

It became clear that accumulating a million bucks—or even my Brand Manager annual salary—wasn't nearly as important as feeling like a million bucks. So I said goodbye to awkward office potlucks, went back to school to study Nutrition, and soon after started my holistic health coaching practice.

Helping people feel better was way more gratifying than strategizing about how to shove more smoked sausages down their throats. But I became discouraged when my clients couldn't consistently reach their goals, and the perfectionist in me wanted to understand why.

It made no sense. I was dishing out sound advice that didn't require diets or deprivation or big sweeping changes. I had clients who were eager to make change and ready to get healthy. They knew exactly what to do and had an expert practically holding their hand every step of the way. Yet, to their great frustration—as well as mine—they often couldn't follow through.

Finally, it hit me! It wasn't my clients who were failing. It was the process. They didn't have the systems and tools they needed to incorporate the changes they so desperately wanted to make into their already crammed schedules. With only so much time in the day, they simply didn't know how or where to squeeze in all the good, healthy stuff.

As the mother of three wild little humans, I know firsthand how hectic life can be. But, despite the frenzied state of my life, I was somehow managing to take good care of both my family and myself. All those organizational and planning skills I'd learned in business school were being put to good use. I was running my life like a boss!

Once I figured out what I was doing right, it was easy to teach my clients how to do the same thing. Just like in the business world, personal success is calculated. Getting healthy isn't just about wanting to look, feel, think, or be better. It's about making a cohesive plan, avoiding pitfalls, and managing your life accordingly.

That's where my *Self-Made Wellionaire* system comes in. It's simple. It's fun. It will change your life!

So let's get down to business.

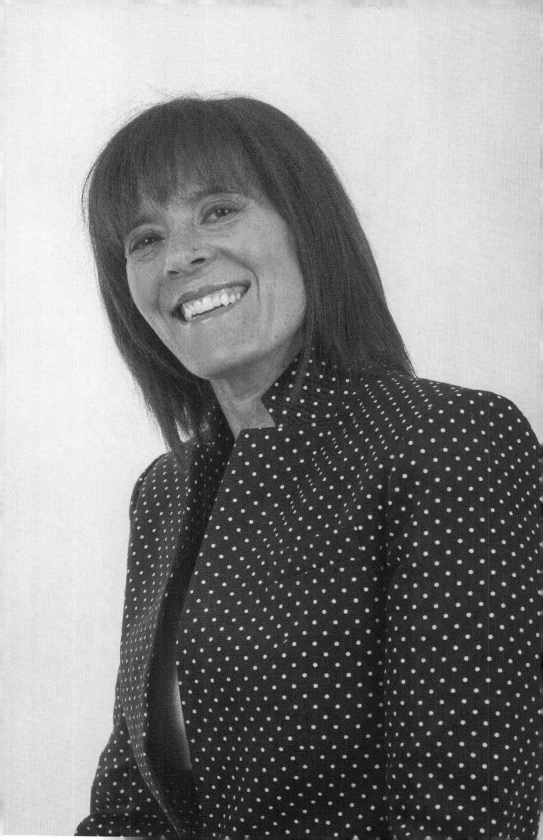

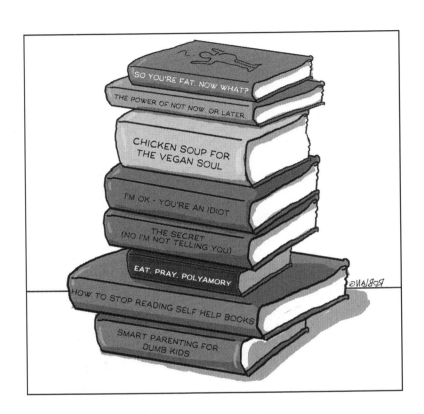

How to Use This Book

By now you probably have a pile of "self help" ~~books~~ coasters collecting dust on your nightstand.

Perhaps you skimmed through them in earnest, hoping they would provide the kick in the pants you so desperately need to stop mismanaging your life. Instead, their platitudes and soft talk coddled you like a toddler, lulling you back to the land of laziness and same old lame excuses. Those books failed to prop you up. Though—bonus!—if you stack your copy of *The Sacred Text on Reawakening Your Cryogenic Dharma* underneath the leg of your wobbly nightstand it might succeed in finally fixing it.

You can read mystical philosophies and abstract advice somewhere else, sometime when you don't have a real life to straighten out. But if you want a book that tells you exactly what you need to do to finally get your shit together and start feeling your best, you're in the right place. This book is practical. It combines the best of what I learned in my MBA program with the best of what I've learned in my holistic health coaching practice.

Part One is all about using basic business strategies to begin planning how you are going to make your wellions. You'll discover how to become the CEO of your life by creating a clear vision, setting achievable goals, and formulating a relevant wellness action plan. This section of the book is packed with hands-on exercises so you can do the work now, instead of putting it off forever.

In Part Two you'll learn how to manage your time, stay accountable, and avoid common pitfalls that could put your riches at risk. Approach these chapters in the manner that best suits your schedule and lifestyle. Digest it like you would your favorite cocktail (or mocktail!)—if you like to nurse your drink, pull it out for about 20 minutes or so to let it really sink in. Or if you're more of a binge drinker, throw it back all at once. Either way, don't forget to actually pay attention and complete the exercises! By the end of the week you'll know how to start planning your self-made wellions and you'll want to give yourself a big, fat raise for being clever enough to buy this little gem. (You can also download all of the exercises on my author website so you can continue to use them in the future.)

Part Three is where the big payoff happens. Chapters 9 to 13 are all about giving you simple strategies for living like a Wellionaire that will teach you how to get out of your own way so you can stop feeling crappy and start feeling radiant. Each chapter is split up into specific lessons, like eating better, exercising, reducing stress, and maximizing your energy, with corresponding action steps that can easily be applied no matter how busy you are. Feel free to read this section in its entirety or skip to the chapter or chapters that are most relevant to your current goals.

Be sure to check out the glossaries at the back of the book for an entertainingly original take on common business phrases and expressions. Pay particular attention to the Wellionaire's Glossary, as this is a rich language you are going to want to learn.

By the time you're done with the book, you'll be the self-healthiest person you know!

PART ONE:

Becoming a Self-Made Wellionaire

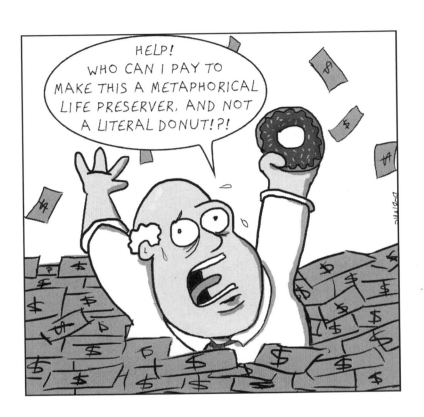

CHAPTER 1

What It Means To Be a Self-Made Wellionaire

Think a business is only as healthy as its bottom line?

In reality, money in the bank doesn't add up to much if a company isn't being managed well.

The same thing goes for you and me. Not only is wealth meaningless if we aren't healthy, true success is impossible.

You might be an executive at a large tech company, but if you've got brain fog from eating junk food all day long you're probably not effective in the boardroom. Likewise, you might live in a beautiful home on Charmed Street and have the most perfect, non-nose-picking kids in the world, but if you're walking around like a zombie all day because your energy is in the toilet, you can't truly enjoy your time together. (And no, you can't pay a plumber to help you.)

That's why more and more of us are discovering that traditional wealth isn't all it's cracked up to be. The best investments have little to do with the price of gold or dead presidents... and everything to do with balance and happiness.

The Definition of **Wellionaire**

To be a Wellionaire you don't need to be sitting on piles of cash, so you can stretch your legs in first class, model the latest fancy handbag, or smear luxurious caviar-infused face cream all over your pores. While having those things can certainly make you feel like a star (and possibly smell like a fish), true success isn't about kickin' it like a Kardashian.

Wellionaires first cultivate an environment in which their brains and bods can function at the highest level. Success naturally follows. It's about what's happening behind the scenes: having energy, minimizing stress, fostering purpose, being fit, and feeling whole.

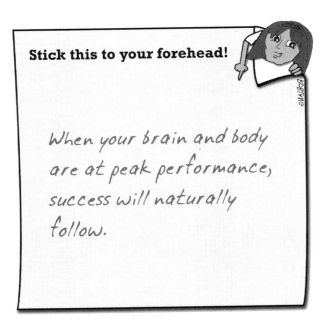

Stick this to your forehead!

When your brain and body are at peak performance, success will naturally follow.

Self-Made

Wellionaires are always self-made because nobody can get healthy for you. It's up to you to step up and start running your life like a boss.

Time and again I've seen this play out with my clients. Those who can create discipline and organization around getting healthy are the ones most likely to rock life—whatever your definition of rockin' life might be—whether you desire to be the next great start-up whiz or you long to give away your worldly possessions so you can get down with your guru in some faraway Ashram.

Ironically, as often as the corporate world may get it wrong, it also holds many of the answers for achieving wellth. Successful managers achieve their goals because they know how to apply a broad range of proven tactics. They take charge, have a vision, set goals, make a plan, take action, manage pitfalls, and create a culture of growth. These business strategies are the same ones you can use to thrive in your personal life.

The first step toward becoming a Wellionaire and leading the life you long for is to think like a manager—and, trust me, the perks are pretty unbeatable.

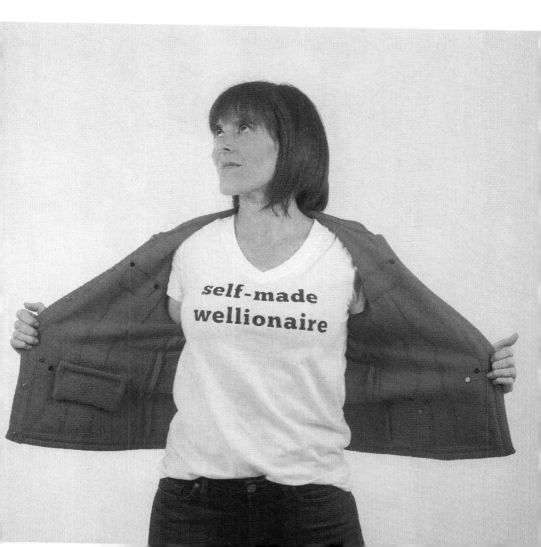

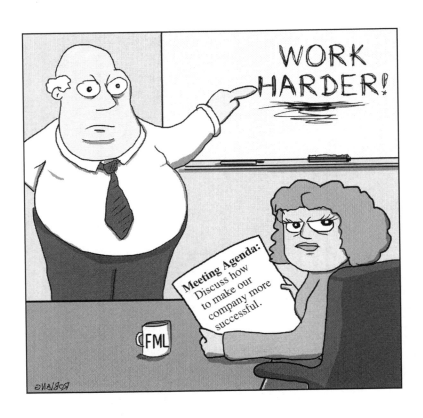

CHAPTER 2

Think Like a (Good) Manager

If I asked you to name an amazing manager you and all your co-workers aspired to be like, you'd probably stare at me like a deer in headlights.

Don't worry.

Your inability to remember your best manager has nothing to do with faulty wiring or a chronic Gingko biloba deficiency, I assure you. It's more likely that you haven't had a really great manager. Many of us haven't.

While average managers may be a dime a dozen, good ones are hard to come by.

In fact, it's quite possible that your last boss made Michael Scott, Steve Carrell's character from *The Office*, look like serious CEO material. Or maybe you had the misfortune of working for the ever-unpopular Mr. Micro-Manager, Ms. Constant Critic, or Mr. Lack of Direction.

Perhaps along the way you even decided you could do the job way better than those clowns.

Well, you're right. You can! If you're reading this book, we'll assume you're the type who takes action and strives for improvement. Even if you have no prior management experience, you are capable of presiding over own self-health with gusto.

Why, then, do so many people suck at it?

Because managing anything well is hard work. It takes total commitment, especially when it comes to self-health. It isn't just a 9-to-5 gig. You can't clock out. You don't get to go on sabbatical. There are no all-expense paid business trips to Miami with Sue, the party animal from Finance. Though, come to think of it, do you really want to risk a reprise of her plastered performance of "These Boobs Were Made for Walking Off the Job" at the next conference? Clever as it was.

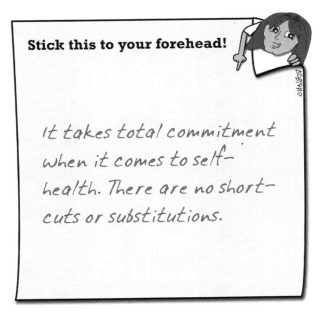

Stick this to your forehead!

It takes total commitment when it comes to self-health. There are no short-cuts or substitutions.

Managing your wellions may not sound like a barrel full of monkeys, but it's a heck of lot more satisfying. Plus it's actually a whole lot easier than it seems.

I'll let you in on the big secret: There are only six things you need to focus on. These are the steps that help superstar managers effectively run businesses, and they are the same simple steps I use to help my clients manage their wellions.

Although we all know how to recognize a bad manager, few know what it really takes to be a successful manager. All you have to do is:

1. Take charge. The best managers and Wellionaires don't sit around waiting for someone else to get things started. They step up and take charge. Hell, they lead the charge. As leaders, good managers reward and recognize quality work, and they encourage and nurture employees. They act decisively. They're firm when needed. And most of all, they know how to inspire and motivate.

2. Have a vision. Understanding that everything is dynamic, great managers and Wellionaires evaluate their business regularly to stay on track. They put the lessons of the past to work, fueled by their hopes for the future, to pinpoint what needs to happen right now. In other words, they formulate a clear vision of what they want to achieve.

3. Organize resources. Skilled managers and Wellionaires know how to prioritize their time, money, and human resources to maximize productivity and capacity. These master delegators can rally their team using a divide-and-conquer strategy to fulfill their most important objectives efficiently. Understanding that their weakness is someone else's strength, they focus on what they know and outsource what they don't.

4. Plan for success. Quality managers and Wellionaires don't just wing it. They use their vision to inspire goals that are SMART: specific, measurable, achievable, relevant and time-bound. Then they carefully construct a feasible action plan that aligns with their goals and follow it to the letter—and they keep an eye on their progress toward those goals.

5. Take action. Effective managers and Wellionaires already know how they are going to execute their plan. So following through and taking action is a no-brainer. Their plan isn't pie-in-the-sky. It's highly achievable and well thought out. But, understanding that no plan is guaranteed, they implement contingency systems and hold themselves accountable to their goals. They direct their efforts toward what can be changed and don't get hung up on things outside their control.

6. Continuously improve. Excellent managers and Wellionaires know that there's always room for improvement. They track and assess their performance to see where they're falling short. Then they fine-tune their tactics accordingly and use the past to help forecast the future.

Using simple systems and guided exercises, I'm going to walk you through exactly what you need to do to start making your wellions. Yes, it takes some effort. But it's worth it!

Becoming a Wellionaire might not land you a private jet or the coveted Black Card. But it comes with its own set of pretty fantastic bonuses. In exchange for working so hard, you'll feel better, think better, and look better.

Whether as a parent, partner, friend, or employee—feeling better makes you function better. Thinking better will make you a more valuable, focused and productive employee—not to mention Sudoku player. And looking better will make you... well... effin' hot.

So here's to becoming an amazing manager of your self-health.

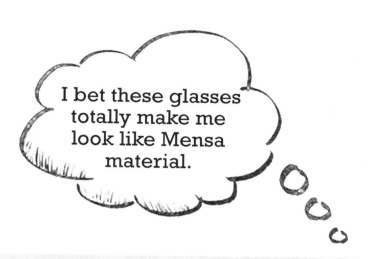

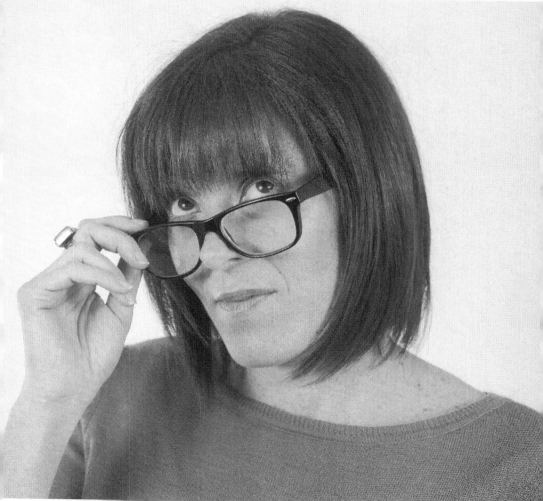

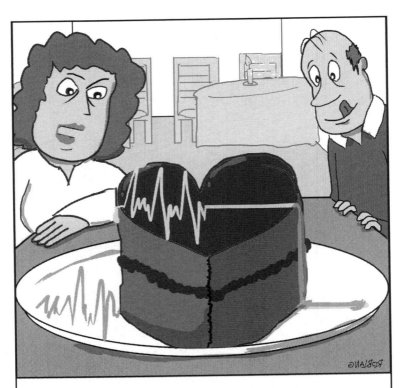

I can't put my finger on it, but something's telling me we should've skipped the berry-drizzled double chocolate heart cake.

CHAPTER 3

Creating Your Wellthy Vision

I have a tendency to wander off and get turned around pretty easily. Shiny objects and tantalizing trinkets sidetrack me.

If not for technological wonders like GPS and Google Maps, I'd be nowhere right now. Or at least nowhere near where I'm supposed to be.

I'm not alone in this. Many people need a compass to guide them where they want to go or they risk being perpetually lost and confused.

It's no different when it comes to wellness. In fact, it's even easier to get off track with self-health goals because there are all sorts of temptations and distractions you're likely to encounter along the way. That's why, whether you're going food shopping or starting a daily exercise regime, having a clear vision is essential.

I don't mean the kind of vision you had back in college after downing a fistful of magic mushrooms or a Venti-sized cup of peyote tea. I'm talking about the type of vision that helps you know which actions and choices will lead you to your desired outcome and propel you forward. Though, if imagining yourself walking over a rainbow bridge made from unicorn horns will keep you motivated, by all means, feel free.

What Is a Vision?

Businesses create vision statements to serve as an aspirational description of what they would like to achieve in the future. For example, Google's vision statement is "to provide access to the world's information in one click." That's no surprise, given that Google's most popular product is its search engine.

Similarly, a personal vision is a broad idea of how you want to look, feel, and be in the future. It goes beyond saying "I want to be healthier" or "I want to manage my time better." A clear vision identifies the change you seek to make and your reason for wanting to make the change and then imagines a better outcome. This understanding motivates and inspires you to achieve your wellness goals.

> With your sights set on your desired outcome, you'll be more willing to stay the course even when things get tough.

When you visualize a preferred scenario you can say to yourself "I want to lose weight because small children keep asking me if I have a baby in my tummy. I'm going to finally get rid of this excess belly fat." Or "I want to get in shape so I can run around with my kids on the playground instead of always watching like a blob from the sidelines." A vision doesn't even need to stretch that far into the future. It can be something as simple as "I want to get in and out of the store quickly so I can get home in time for kick-off. I'm not going to waste time perusing end-cap displays of cake baking supplies when I need a cake like I need a hole in the head. I am going to stay focused on grabbing only the four items I need."

See the difference?

With your sights set on your desired outcome, you'll be more willing to stay the course even when things get tough. This is how the best managers develop their employees. They don't just think about what is, they visualize what could be.

A vision is about seeing the big picture. You can't set realistic wellness goals unless you're clear about what needs to change and where you hope to see yourself in the future.

Easier said than done!

Sometimes it can be overwhelming to figure out what you want your future to look like.

The good news is you already know what needs to change. These are the things that keep you up at night. They resurface. They make you insecure.

"The doctor said I'm at risk for heart disease."

"I'm chronically constipated."

"I'm fatigued all the time and can't get through the day without napping."

"I'm officially obese."

If only I could fix it.

Luckily you can, as long as you have a clear vision!

How to Formulate Your Vision

1. Identify the change(s) you most want to make. It's tempting to try to totally overhaul everything about yourself at once. Why not lose ten pounds, learn how to zonk out for eight hours straight, supercharge your energy and consistently start flossing your teeth with seaweed?

All. Right. Now.

Appealing as it may be, that's a terrible idea.

Making any kind of self-healthy change is a big deal. That's why a blanket approach simply doesn't work. Instead, when creating your vision, focus on one key area at a time and you'll be much more likely to succeed. Choose your highest wellness priority carefully, because it's where you will dedicate most of your resources for the next three to six months.

2. Ask yourself "Why do I want to make this change?" It's not enough to say "I want to lose weight" or "I want to feel energized." You need to know why you want to lose weight or have more energy. The "why" is going to help shape your vision and keep you motivated to accomplish your goals.

Examples:
- I want to eat better because I'm tired of feeling like a walking medicine cabinet.
- I want to be more regular because I'm sick of pooping once a week and feeling bloated.
- I want to start exercising more because I'm tired of stuffing my flabby body into my clothes and feeling uncomfortable.
- I want to have more energy because I'm sick of dozing off in meetings and I'm worried I'm going to get canned.

Notice how your "I want to" statement is directly connected to the adverse results you are experiencing. Be real with yourself about the negative impact of your behavior in this step. It's not the time to be gentle. We'll put a more positive spin on things in the next step.

3. Envision a better outcome. This is where things start to get a little rosier, as you tap into your dreams, hopes, and aspirations. You have to put yourself in your future shoes and imagine what you want your circumstances to look like down the road.

Examples:
- I see myself medication-free with my cholesterol and blood pressure under control
- I see myself feeling lighter and having one good bowel movement a day.
- I see myself fitting comfortably into my clothes and feeling secure wearing the styles I like.
- I see myself waking up feeling alert and naturally being able to stay energized throughout the entire day.

Notice how your "I see myself" statement is more positive than your "I want to" statement as you begin to connect the change you seek to make with your desired outcome.

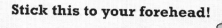

Stick this to your forehead!

Three to six months is a good timeframe to work with when envisioning what you want to be, do or look like. It gives you a large enough window to imagine the impact of your changes and a realistic amount of time to develop healthy new habits.

4. Identify potential pitfalls. In the business world, a SWOT analysis is often used to organize a company's thinking and better understand the environment in which they are trying to accomplish goals. SWOT is an acronym that stands for strengths, weaknesses, opportunities, and threats. It's also a helpful tool for individuals when organizing their wellness vision.

Start by asking yourself four questions and remember to keep it B.S.-free:

1. *What are my related strengths?* These are the skills and capabilities that are going to help you in achieving your goals.

2. *What are my related weaknesses?* These are the skills and capabilities you lack that could prevent you from achieving your goal.

3. *What opportunities do I see for improvement in the future?* These are the moments that are going to help you grow so you can fully realize your goals.

4. *What are the threats that could prevent me from achieving my goal?*

These are the factors that could derail you from fully realizing your desires.

Example 1—Andy: *I want to eat better because I'm tired of feeling like a walking medicine cabinet. I see myself medication-free with my cholesterol and blood pressure under control.*

What are my related strengths?
- I enjoy healthy foods when I manage to eat them.
- I'm an adventurous eater and even tried cuttlefish once (then promptly vomited—but still).

What are my related weaknesses?
- I'm an awful cook.
- I eat a lot of meals out, especially work lunches.
- When I eat out, I tend to order the heavier items on the menu—all at the same time.

What opportunities do I see for improvement in the future?
- Learning how to cook something that doesn't go in the microwave.
- Making better choices when eating out.

What are the threats that could prevent me from achieving my goal?
- I'm a consultant and I travel a lot for work. The airport is my home away from home. I even know the TSA agents by name.
- When I'm home I crave comfort food, like the triple bacon pizza from Sal's, and since I don't have time to go grocery shopping I eat whatever's easy.

Example 2—Maria: *I want to be more regular because I'm sick of pooping once a week and feeling bloated. I see myself feeling lighter and having one good bowel movement a day.*

What are my related strengths?
- I enjoy lots of fruits and veggies.
- I have a Costco-size package of toilet paper just waiting at the ready.

What are my related weaknesses?

- I have a hard time giving up foods I love even if I know they're hurting me.
- My middle name might as well be Dairy.

What opportunities do I see for improvement in the future?

- Eliminating foods that are messing with my digestion and shutting down the fart factory.
- Finding substitutes for the foods I will miss the most.

What are the threats that could prevent me from achieving my goal?

- The rest of my family members don't have food sensitivities and my kids don't like change.
- Lasagna. Enchiladas. Omelets. Pretty much everything I cook for my family has cheese in it. I'm worried that I won't have the willpower to cook something separate for me, and I don't have time to prepare multiple meals to try to please everyone.

Example 3—Carol: *I want to start exercising more because I'm tired of stuffing my flabby body into my clothes and feeling uncomfortable. I see myself fitting comfortably into my clothes and feeling secure wearing the styles I like.*

What are my related strengths?

- I like to be active and enjoy taking the kids hiking and swimming. With the exception of the time I went to hot yoga and nearly passed out in a cesspool of someone else's sweat, I like to try out new fitness classes.

What are my related weaknesses?

- I have a tight budget and a crazy schedule that makes it hard to go to the gym.
- I snack all day long and might possibly kill for Nacho Cheese Doritos.

What opportunities do I see for improvement in the future?

- Learning quick, effective exercises that I can do anytime, anywhere.

- Blocking out time in my schedule to exercise so that nothing interferes.
- Finding some healthier snack options that don't leave a layer of orange dust on my fingers.

What are the threats that could prevent me from achieving my goal?
- I'm a single mom who works 10 hours a day and then has to cook dinner and help my school-age kids with their homework. Did I mention it's Calculus?
- I have an (aforementioned) daytime Doritos addiction and nightly ice cream habit that won't quit, not to mention a stash of Halloween candy that I may have "borrowed" from my kids.

Example 4—Peter: I want to have more energy because I'm sick of dozing off in meetings and I'm worried I'm going to get canned. I see myself waking up feeling alert and naturally being able to stay energized throughout the entire day.

What are my related strengths?
- I like to sleep. A lot.
- I'm typically home at a reasonable time. Except for my weekly Thursday night dart league events. Then all bets are off.

What are my related weaknesses?
- I watch TV until the wee hours of the morning.
- I often wake up in the middle of the night thinking about work projects.

What opportunities do I see for improvement in the future?
- Going to bed earlier.
- Learning how to be more Zen.

What are the threats that could prevent me from achieving my goal?
- I'm single and pretty much married to my television. I regularly binge on Netflix and often fall asleep on the couch.
- Work is super stressful and I've always got a big deadline looming. It's hard for me to turn off my brain and just relax, unless I'm distracted by "Cheryl." It's normal to name your TV, right?

Your Turn: Create Your Vision

Now it's your turn. Don't put this exercise off. Don't kid yourself and say you're going to come back to it. Do. It. Now. You can download a copy of this template at **JillGinsberg.com/templates.**

Step 1: Write down the one or two wellness changes you most want to make in the next three to six months.

Change 1: _____

Change 2 (optional): _____

Step 2: List the most important reason why you want to make the change. This is the basis of your whole vision. Begin with the phrase "I want to <Insert Your Answer to Change 1 here> because _____."

I want to _____

because _____

_____

Step 3: Now imagine the intended outcome you hope to achieve in three to six months' time. This is likely the opposite of how you are feeling now. Begin with the phrase "I see myself _____."

I see myself _____

_____

Step 4: Answer the SWOT questions on the next page to identify the trouble point that threatens to derail you from succeeding. Make sure your answers directly relate to your responses in steps 1 and 2.

STRENGTHS: What are my related strengths?	WEAKNESSES: What are my related weaknesses?
OPPORTUNITIES: What opportunities do I see for improvement in the future?	THREATS: What are the threats that could prevent me from achieving my goal?

Step 5. Connect the dots by putting steps 1 through 4 together and—boom!—you have a clear, SWOT tested vision that will help you to formulate your goals and action steps. Taking the extra time now to write out a cohesive vision is well worth it. It is your roadmap for how to—and how not to—start on the path to becoming a Self-Made Wellionaire, and you will want to refer back to it many times over.

Sample Vision 1—Andy:

The doctor said I'm at risk for heart disease. I want to start eating better because I'm tired of feeling like a walking medicine cabinet. I see myself medication-free with my cholesterol and blood pressure under control.

I'm an adventurous eater and enjoy healthy foods. But I eat a lot of meals out, especially work lunches, and tend to order too much unhealthy food. I don't know how to cook and am afraid I will set the whole kitchen on fire if I so much as look at my toaster.

I need to make better choices when I eat out and travel. And I want to learn how to cook some basic healthy foods and keep healthy options on hand so I don't just go for whatever's fast and easy.

Sample Vision 2—Carol:

I'm officially obese. I want to start exercising more because I'm tired of stuffing my flabby body into my clothes and feeling uncomfortable. I see myself fitting comfortably into my clothes and feeling secure wearing the styles I like.

I like to be active, enjoy taking the kids hiking and swimming, and like to try out new fitness classes. But I have a tight budget and a crazy schedule that make it hard to go to the gym. I get easily bored with most types of exercise, and I snack all day long.

I need to find quick, effective exercises that even a single mom who works 10 hours a day can do anytime, anywhere. I also need to block out time in my schedule to exercise so that nothing interferes. And I need to find some healthier snack options other than what's in the vending machine.

My Vision:

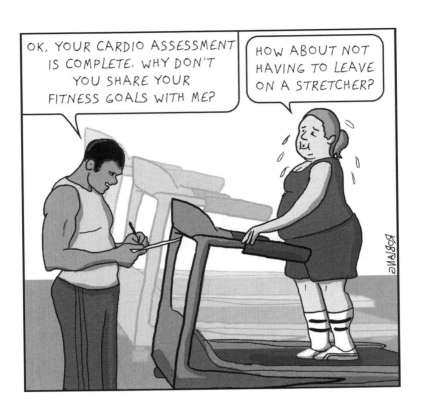

CHAPTER 4

How to Set SMARTy-Pants Goals

Businesses regularly set annual goals to direct and motivate employees, facilitate planning, and establish a benchmark to gauge and evaluate success.

Individuals set goals for the same reasons. Whether your objective is to land a fat promotion next year, become a (gasp!) vegan, or finally fix that damn leaky faucet, your goals act as a roadmap—they direct you where you want to go and remind you how to get there when times get tough.

Goals are especially important when you're looking to become a Wellionaire. When you set a goal to run your first half-marathon and, by your second week of training, all you want to do is curl up in the fetal position and scribble DO NOT DISTURB on your forehead in indelible Sharpie, your goals hold you accountable and make you more likely to get back up off your ass(et) so you can keep logging those miles.

How to Define Your Goals

Now that you have a clear vision and you understand why you want to become self-healthy, it's time to set more specific goals to accomplish over the next three to six months. Your goals are more specific than your vision and tell you what you need to do in order to achieve your desired outcome.

Setting your goals helps you organize your thinking and makes it easier to identify the action steps necessary to meet your wellness objectives, which we will do in the next chapter.

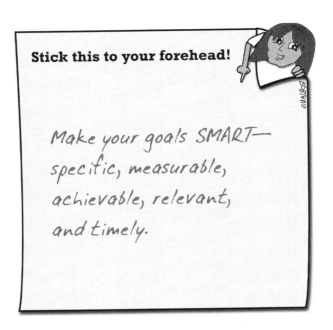

Stick this to your forehead!

Make your goals SMART— specific, measurable, achievable, relevant, and timely.

There are five strategies for setting effective wellness goals:

1. Make them SMART. Businesses often rely on a proven system called SMART to help create well-defined goals, such as "create four new product features in 2016," "achieve a customer satisfaction rating of 95 percent by the second quarter" and "reduce our cost of goods by $1.25 per unit in the next six months."

SMART is an acronym that stands for:

> **A. Specific:** Your goals should state as clearly as possible what you hope to achieve. There's no room for ambiguity. Ask yourself "What exactly do I want to accomplish?" An example of a specific wellness goal is "By the end of 2015 I will be able to consistently stay awake every day for 12 hours straight without needing to depend on coffee, Red Bull, or smelling salts."

Or "Starting one week from today I will begin eating balanced meals consisting of 33.3 percent carbs, 33.3 percent healthy fats and 33.3 percent lean protein. Except for Sunday brunch, which will consist of 100% Bloody Mary's.

B. Measurable: Your goals should have a quantifiable outcome or "success metric" that allows you to know with certainty whether or not you've accomplished your objective. This might be pounds, inches, glasses of water, or some other quantifiable variable that lets you track your progress. Ask yourself "How will I know when I've achieved this goal?"

For instance, if your goal is "Instead of hitting the drive-thru on my way to work, I will eat three healthy homemade breakfasts per week for the next eight weeks" then by the end of the week it's going to be pretty clear whether or not you lived up to your end of the deal. Bonus: The fellas at the office might finally stop calling you Mr. McSausage Breath.

C. Achievable: Your goals should help you grow and stretch while still being attainable. Ask yourself "Is this a realistic and achievable goal for where I am in life right now?"

For example, I would love to learn how to sing like Adele but there ain't no way in hell that's happening in this lifetime. However, figuring out how to master "Twinkle, Twinkle Little Star" on my toddler's miniature piano may be possible.

D. Relevant: Your goals should move you down your desired path and match the outcome you are working toward. Anything that takes you in a different direction from your vision isn't relevant right now. Ask yourself "Does my goal match the outcome I am seeking?"

For instance, if your objective is to reduce anxiety and you have a phobia of heights then having a goal of "Before my 40th birthday I will ride on every ferris wheel in the United States" isn't exactly aligned with that, whereas something associated with deep breathing likely would be.

E. Timely: Your goals should have a definitive end date with a specific stated outcome at the conclusion of the goal. Ask yourself "When do I hope to accomplish this goal?" The endpoint of your goal should never be so far away that it seems unattainable.

For example, if your goal is "I will have six-pack abs in time for my high school reunion in three years" you can bet you're going to lose focus well before the big event. Remember to keep your timeframe relatively short, ideally looking three to six months ahead.

2. **Break up goals to help keep you on track.** Breaking up goals into smaller chunks or mini goals makes them feel less intimidating and more achievable. It makes mountains feel like hills. Or a D cup feel like an A cup. For instance, "lose 12 pounds in three months" becomes "lose four pounds per month," which then becomes "lose one pound per week." Or "try four healthy new superfoods this month" becomes "try one new superfood per week." Breaking up your goals also makes it easier to continuously track your progress.

3. **Write down your goals.** The moment you write down your goal, it becomes more tangible. You declare your intention and set your wellth in motion, even before you take your first step. Putting your goals in writing helps clarify thinking and compels action. Being able to refer back to your written goals also allows you to track your progress so you can see just how far you've really gone, even when it feels like you're moving in slow motion.

4. **State your goals in the positive.** Phrasing your goals in a positive way allows you to focus on the productive changes you want to make rather than on the negative behaviors you are seeking to change. For example, instead of saying "I don't want to be a picky eater" you can say "Over the next six weeks, I will expand my eating repertoire by discovering four healthy new foods to regularly incorporate into my diet." Or instead of saying "I don't want to be a permanent fixture on my couch anymore" you can say "I will add 30 minutes of movement to my day starting December 1."

5. **Start from where you are.** Each of us is different, and we all have varying nutritional and physical needs that are dependent on our personal tastes and preferences, activity level, age, blood types, metabolic rate, food tolerances, stress level, activity level, and genetic background, among other variables.

So you can't base your goals around keeping up with your best friend, who may be a former 200-meter track star. Or your neighbor who may smoke two packs of reefer cigarettes a day.

The key is to set yourself up for success by focusing on your own vision of wellth. Not somebody else's.

If you've never swam a day in your life outside of the shallow end, it's not wise to throw on your Speedo and head right out on a six-mile deepwater swim with your triathlon-training brother-in-law. If by some miracle you don't drown, your body and ego will both be sore the next day. It makes more sense to start off by getting your feet wet. Then increase your exertion and ramp up the distance as you gain strength and stamina.

Likewise, if you've never eaten a vegetable that didn't come from a can, don't set a goal of drinking a green smoothie for breakfast and eating a kale salad for lunch every day. Start by including one small serving of fresh veggies in your daily diet and make that a consistent habit.

6. **Go for the low-hanging fruit.** I often encourage my clients to set some early goals that are almost guaranteed. In the business world this is referred to as "low hanging fruit," and it essentially means going for the quick win first.

It's good to set some initial "gimme" goals that are easily within your grasp—goals you barely need to stretch to reach, such as "I will drink an extra 8 oz. glass of water per day" or "I will try two new healthy gluten-free grains in the next four weeks." Going for the low-hanging fruit early on gives your confidence a healthy boost so you can then start to stretch more for the stuff that's a little harder to reach.

Other Considerations When Setting Goals

There are a few other important points of consideration when setting your wellness goals:

- *Some things can't be changed.* You won't be doing yourself any good if you try to attack a problem that's not solvable. Just like in business, it's helpful to think about things as either fixed or variable. Weight, for instance, is variable. It can change over time and you often have a fair amount of control over it. Height, on the other hand, is fixed. Once you've stopped growing there's nothing you're going to be able to do to change how tall you are, Mr. "I'm 5'8... AND A HALF INCHES." So remember to go after the stuff that can be altered and learn to live with the stuff that can't.

- *Manage your own expectations.* Otherwise known as "under promise, over deliver." If your goal is to get back to your pre-pregnancy weight and you want to actually keep the extra weight off, you should expect it to take some time. If your goal is to overhaul your eating lifestyle for the long-term, it's going to take a while to learn how to shop, meal plan, and cook accordingly. Set yourself up for success by not being overly aggressive with your expectations while still pushing yourself beyond your comfort zone. If your idea of a vegetable is iceberg lettuce, you don't want to promise to suddenly start bathing your tongue in raw, fermented sauerkraut and *sprouts! sprouts! sprouts!* all day long and then beat yourself up when you can't live up to it. Instead, start by swapping out your iceberg for some spinach.

- *Small shifts are best.* It may feel like taking shortcuts is the fastest way to get places sometimes. But baby steps, although slower, are far more sustainable when it comes to making self-healthy change. Small steps will get you to your goal faster than big leaps because you won't ever take any steps backward. The important thing is, even if you're taking baby steps, you're moving forward in the right direction.

When Should You Reevaluate Your Goals?

Businesses typically set goals annually in preparation for the start of their fiscal year. Many companies then review their goals in depth on a quarterly basis and make adjustments as needed.

I also like to apply this annual/quarterly approach toward evaluating and updating personal goals. The time period is long enough to make meaningful progress toward your goals but short enough so that you can maintain your focus. By reviewing your personal goals at the start of every quarter, you can adjust to seasonal changes that impact your activities, behavior, and lifestyle.

There may be other occasions when it will also be appropriate to evaluate and adjust your goals. Whenever you experience upheaval (no, the season finale of your favorite television show doesn't count) or a major life transition, job change, divorce, injury, or significant change to your home life, you want to take a moment to reevaluate your goals with fresh eyes and, where necessary, modify them to better suit your changed circumstances.

Your Turn: Create SMART Goals

Now it's time for you to create some goals of your own! Here's how:

1. Your vision statement will help you to formulate your goals. Review it and identify anything that could be a goal.

EXAMPLE 1—Andy

Vision:

The doctor said I'm at risk for heart disease. I want to start eating better because I'm tired of feeling like a walking medicine cabinet. I see myself medication-free with my cholesterol and blood pressure under control.

I'm an adventurous eater and enjoy healthy foods. But I eat a lot of meals out, especially work lunches, and tend to order too much unhealthy food. I don't know how to cook and am afraid I will set the whole kitchen on fire if I so much as look at my toaster.

I need to make better choices when I eat out and travel. And I want to learn how to cook some basic healthy foods and keep healthy options on hand so I don't just go for whatever's fast and easy.

Possible Goals:
- Lower cholesterol
- Lower blood pressure
- Learn how to cook
- Eat healthier at work and when I travel
- Shop for healthy groceries

EXAMPLE 2—Carol

Vision:

I'm officially obese. I want to lose weight because I'm tired of stuffing my flabby body into my clothes and feeling uncomfortable. I see myself comfortably fitting into my clothes and feeling secure wearing the styles I like.

I like to be active, enjoy taking the kids hiking and swimming, and like to try out new fitness classes. But I have a tight budget and a crazy schedule that make it hard to go to the gym. I get easily bored with most types of exercise, and I snack all day long.

I need to find quick, effective exercises that even a single mom who works 10 hours a day can do anytime, anywhere. I also need to block out time in my schedule to exercise so that nothing interferes. And I need to find some healthier snack options other than what's in the vending machine.

Possible Goals:
- Lose weight
- Exercise more
- Find quick, effective exercises that I can do anywhere
- Schedule exercise
- Find healthier snack options

Now that you've seen a couple of examples, enter your Vision from Chapter 3 on the next page. Then, in the section provided underneath, list any possible goals you have identified. You can download a copy of this template at **jillginsberg.com/templates.**

My Vision:

_____
_____
_____
_____
_____
_____
_____
_____

Possible Goals:

- _____
- _____
- _____
- _____
- _____
- _____
- _____
- _____
- _____
- _____
- _____

2. Then turn your possible goals into SMART goals that are specific, measurable, achievable, relevant, and timely.

Vision Example 1—Andy:

The doctor said I'm at risk for heart disease. I want to start eating better because I'm tired of feeling like a walking medicine cabinet. I see myself medication-free with my cholesterol and blood pressure under control. I'm an adventurous eater and enjoy healthy foods. But I eat a lot of meals out, especially work lunches, and tend to order too much unhealthy food. I don't know how to cook and am afraid I will set the whole kitchen on fire if I so much as look at my toaster.

I need to make better choices when I eat out and travel. And I want to learn how to cook some basic healthy foods and keep healthy options on hand so I don't just go for whatever's fast and easy.

Possible Goals Turned into SMART Goals:
- Lower cholesterol: I will lower my LDL cholesterol by 10 percent in the next 90 days.
- Lower blood pressure: Within six months I will have a blood pressure reading of 120 over 80.
- Learn how to cook: I will learn how to cook one new healthy meal per week for the next three months.
- Eat healthier at work and when I travel: I will eat a healthy, balanced work lunch every day for the next 30 days.
- Shop for healthy groceries: 80 percent of the groceries I purchase each week will consist of fruits, veggies, and other whole foods.

Vision Example 2—Carol:

I'm officially obese. I want to lose weight because I'm tired of stuffing my flabby body into my clothes and feeling uncomfortable all day. I see myself comfortably fitting into my clothes and feeling secure wearing the styles I like.

I like to be active, enjoy taking the kids hiking and swimming, and like to try out new fitness classes. But I have a tight budget and a crazy schedule that make it hard to go to the gym. I get easily bored with most types of exercise, and I snack all day long.

I need to find quick, effective exercises that even a single mom who works 10 hours a day can do anytime, anywhere. I also need to block out time in my schedule to exercise so that nothing interferes. And I need to find some healthier snack options other than what's in the vending machine.

Possible Goals Turned into SMART Goals:
- Lose weight: I will lose 12 pounds in 12 weeks.
- Exercise more: I will exercise 30 minutes three days per week for the next ten weeks.
- Find quick, effective exercises that I can do anywhere: Within four weeks I will identify two to three forms of exercise that are quick, effective, and free. Couch squats anyone?

- Schedule exercise: I will add 30 minutes of movement to each weekday for three months.
- Find healthier snack options: For the next month, I will try two new healthy snack options per week.

Now that you've seen a couple of examples, try turning your possible goals into well-defined SMART goals. Remember to keep the tips provided throughout this chapter in mind.

POSSIBLE GOALS	SMART GOALS
Possible Goal 1:	
Possible Goal 2:	
Possible Goal 3:	
Possible Goal 4:	
Possible Goal 5:	
Possible Goal 6:	

It's best to break your SMART goals down into one-month, three-month, and six-month mini-goals. Using the template provided, go ahead and assign two of your SMART goals to each time period.

SMART GOALS FORM

Write in a start date and an end date. If your goal doesn't have an end date, and it's a self-healthy habit you want to continue, leave that section blank.

You can download a copy of this template at **jillginsberg.com/ templates.**

One month: A single month will sneak up on you fast so be sure to set achievable, low-hanging fruit goals that you can accomplish quickly.

1._____

_____

Start Date:_____   End Date:_____

2. _____

_____

Start Date:_____   End Date:_____

Three months: You have ample time to complete these goals so push yourself out of your comfort zone a bit and give yourself something to reach for.

1._____

_____

Start Date:_____   End Date:_____

2. _____

_____

Start Date:_____   End Date:_____

Six months: In six months, it's possible to create almost any healthy new lifestyle habit, so really try to imagine the possibilities.

1._____

_____

Start Date:_____   End Date:_____

2. _____

_____

Start Date:_____   End Date:_____

Once You've Achieved Your Goals

Once you've achieved your goals it's important to check in with yourself. Here are a few tips you'll want to remember once you complete your first round of wellness goals:

- **Take the time to celebrate your accomplishments!** Notice how much progress you've made toward your wellthy goals. If the goal was a significant one, reward yourself. You deserve it! Get some new workout gear. Go out to a healthy, new restaurant. Hit the naked spa for some TLC. Hell, take a vacation day and do it all at the same time!
- **Set new goals!** Remember the continuous improvement concept from Chapter 2? Great managers know that there's always room to improve. Think about what you can tackle next. If you hit your goal weight, maybe you'd like to drop a few more pounds. If you increased your energy, maybe now you can picture yourself signing up for that action-packed spin class you've always wanted to take (your body will thank you! your crotch, not so much).
- **Be honest with yourself!** If you achieved your goal too easily, make your follow up goals more challenging.

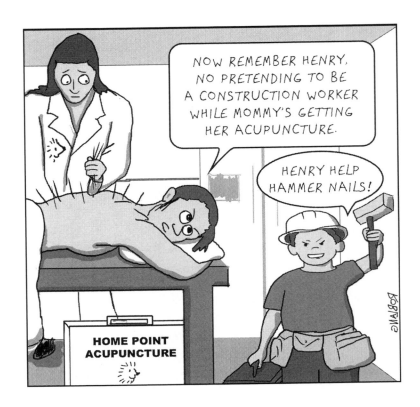

CHAPTER 5

Biz Planning for Success

Creating goals is easy for most managers. The execution is where they flounder. Bad managers don't plan; they react.

While they're busily executing a *ready! fire! aim!* approach, a competitor sneaks through the back door and steals half their market share. The manager is then left scrambling to respond to sudden revenue losses, missed financial targets, and a barrage of unpleasant middle-finger pointing.

As a Wellionaire, you need to carefully construct an action plan for success so you can accurately hit your goals. Flying by the seat of your yoga pants won't get you very far. If your goal is to reduce stress it's not wise to randomly plop yourself down in the middle of your kitchen floor and begin chanting, as you wait for your chakras to start vibrating in resonance with the universe. The only thing you're liable to become more mindful of is the dust bunny under the fridge.

Before you jump in and start trying to reduce your stress willy nilly, you first want to come up with a strategy and then devise some simple action steps. If your strategy for lowering stress is to try meditating, you might begin by researching basic meditation techniques, blocking out some alone time, finding a quiet, comfy spot, and maybe even downloading one of those handy guided meditation podcasts... ahhhhh, it's like pure Xanax spewing from the speakers.

Lots of well-intentioned people are great at dreaming about what they'd like to accomplish. They get so excited about the prospect of becoming a Wellionaire that they immediately want to start setting their goals into motion, but they forget about the importance of creating an action plan. Ultimately, they fail.

If you've already done the hard work of drafting a clear vision and designing your goals, creating an action plan is a simple process that only requires you to invest a few extra minutes—and the ROI is unbeatable!

How to Create an Action Plan

The SMART goals you worked so hard to create in the previous chapter are an awesome start. But now you need an action plan so you can begin to effectively and successfully tackle them.

Your action plan breaks your goals down into steps, outlines the resources needed to achieve them, and identifies a timeline for when specific tasks need to be completed.

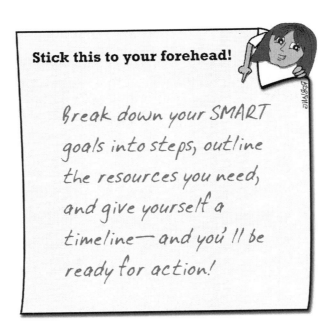

Stick this to your forehead!

Break down your SMART goals into steps, outline the resources you need, and give yourself a timeline—and you'll be ready for action!

There are four basic steps to creating an action plan. Start with a one-month goal and then continue to use this system to accomplish your three-month and six-month goals:

1. **Pick a strategy.** A strategy is a method or plan chosen to bring about your desired goal. The strategy you select will influence the action steps that follow.

   ### What's the difference between strategies and action steps?

   Strategies and action steps are not the same. Managers craft a strategy to achieve a goal, then they execute a series of action steps (often referred to as tactics in the business world) to implement their strategy. Your strategy tells you more about what you want to accomplish, while your action steps tell you how you are going to accomplish your plan.

   For example, to achieve the goal of "increasing inline skate sales by 150 percent by March 2017," management may adopt a strategy of pursuing a new market. To implement that strategy, the company will have to develop the right action steps, which might include manufacturing inline skates for dogs since (duh!) four legs are better than two. Additional action steps might include creating promotional tools for pet stores and increasing their liability insurance for all the lawsuits that are bound to pour in when furry friends everywhere start rolling into oncoming traffic.

   When it comes to wellness, the same critical distinction between strategies and action steps applies. Not wanting to get cavities is a goal. Better hygiene is the strategy for achieving your goal. Flossing is an action step to accomplish your strategy.

   Or you may have a goal of "losing 7 pounds in 7 weeks." But until you know your strategy, you won't know which action steps you want to implement. For instance, if your weight loss strategy is centered around changing your diet, your action steps are going to look way different than your mom's, given that her strategy is to shed those extra holiday pounds by exercising more. Like mom said, "It's not as if those leftover peppermint sugar snowmen cookies are going to eat themselves!"

Regardless of the approach you choose, you want to pursue only one primary goal at a time and then select your strategies accordingly. This is going to help you focus on fulfilling your most important goal.

Different strategies will lead to very different action steps.
The strategy you select to accomplish your goals will greatly impact the action steps you take.

When thinking about your strategy, the key question you want to ask yourself is "How am I going to accomplish my goal?"

Pick a strategy that feels approachable to you. Often this will be the one that you are most excited to try or the one that is best suited to your lifestyle and personality.

In the Implementation section of the book, there is a list of recommended strategies for each wellness lesson, including healthy eating, lifestyle strategies, weight loss strategies, stress reduction strategies, and energy maximization strategies. You will have the option of choosing from the recommended strategies or coming up with your own strategy.

Here are some examples of possible strategies that could be executed for the sample SMART goals outlined in Chapter 4.

- **Goal 1:** Within six months I will have a blood pressure reading of 120 over 80.
  Possible strategies to reduce blood pressure: Reduce sodium consumption; increase exercise; reduce alcohol consumption; eat more fruits; eat more veggies.

- **Goal 2:** Within 90 days I will make Dr. Oz proud and take one solid dump a day.
  Possible strategies to improve elimination: Consume more foods that are good for my digestion; eliminate foods that are slowing down my digestion; drink a mug of my dad's super-potent butt-exploding coffee, also known as "Cup O' Laxative."

- **Goal 3:** I will lose 12 pounds in 12 weeks.
  Possible strategies for weight loss: Exercise more; add in healthier foods; remove unhealthy foods; track consumption.

- **Goal 4:** Within 30 days I will increase my ranking by 2 points on Jill's Magical Energy Scale (which you will learn more about in Chapter 9.)
  Possible strategies for increasing energy: Increase sleep; increase energizing foods; reduce draining foods; reduce stress; improve self-care.

2. **Create your action steps.** For each strategy, you should devise approximately three action steps. You will use your action steps to help implement your strategy and achieve your wellness goals.

Perhaps your goal is to "lose 12 lbs in 12 weeks" and your strategy is to start running. So you decide to keep yourself motivated by signing up for the upcoming "Boob Sweat and Beers" 5K race. Some of your action steps might include: (a) research local races, (b) coerce a friend into joining you, (c) buy a new pair of running shoes, (d) print out a training schedule, and (e) start using it!

The same approach applies to any goal; it doesn't have to be wellness related. For example, if your goal is to purchase a new hot tub, some of your action steps might include: (a) research hot tub manufacturers, (b) hire an electrician, (c) install a pad, (d) schedule delivery, and (e) install some (oops!) privacy fencing so your neighbor's don't have to see that again.

Your action steps should be specific.

As is the case with your goals, in order for your action steps to be effective they also need to be specific. Here are some examples of not-so-specific action steps:

- I will eat a rainbow. (Umm, are you planning on tossing back a jumbo bag of Skittles or eating something that doesn't include nine varieties of artificial coloring?)
- I will run with Jen at work. (What a coincidence! I was thinking of running away with Bob from Finance.)

- I will eat more veggies. (After your soul has departed? Or in this lifetime? And how much is "more"?)

Here are some examples of action steps that are specific and effective:
- I will eat four colorful servings of fruits and veggies every day.
- I will jog with Jen two days per week on our lunch break.
- I will include a veggie at dinner each evening.

Below you can see several sample combinations of goals, strategies, and action steps.

GOAL: Within six months I will have a blood pressure reading of 120 over 80.			
Strategy:	Action Step 1	Action Step 2	Action Step 3
Eat More Fresh Fruits	Add 1/2 cup of fresh berries to my cereal each morning.	Bring a fresh piece of fruit to work to eat as a snack every day.	Drink a fresh fruit smoothie every day.

GOAL: Within 90 days I will make Dr. Oz proud and take one solid dump a day.			
Strategy:	Action Step 1	Action Step 2	Action Step 3
Consume More Things That Are Good For My Digestion	Eat 2 fiber rich foods per day.	Take a probiotic.	Drink five 8 oz. glasses of water per day.

GOAL: I will exercise 30 minutes three days per week for the next 10 weeks.			
Strategy:	Action Step 1	Action Step 2	Action Step 3
Exercise At Home	Clear the clothing and other random debris off of my stationary bike so I can use it for its intended purpose.	Identify three new forms of exercise that are quick, effective, and free. Couch squats, anyone?	Set my alarm for 30 minutes earlier once per week so I have time to do my workout.

Notice how your fitness-related action steps change depending on whether your strategy is to exercise at work or home.

GOAL: I will add 30 minutes of movement to each weekday for three months.			
Strategy: :	Action Step 1	Action Step 2	Action Step 3
Move More At Work	Walk with Mary from HR for 20 minutes during lunch.	Use the stairs instead of the elevator.	During bio-breaks, walk to the farthest bathroom on my floor. Bonus: Nobody will know I stunk it up!

GOAL: Within 30 days I will increase my ranking by 2 points on Jill's Magical Energy Scale.			
Strategy:	Action Step 1	Action Step 2	Action Step 3
Get More Sleep	Turn off all electronics by 8 p.m.	Get in bed at 10 PM every night.	Create a calming bedtime ritual.

GOAL: I will eat a healthy, balanced lunch every day for the next 30 days.			
Strategy:	Action Step 1	Action Step 2	Action Step 3
Have a plan before lunch, whether I've packed a lunch or pre-selected something healthy off the menu	Take a healthy lunch to work on M, W, and F.	Prepare my lunch the night before so I don't forget.	Bring a healthy snack to eat before my Tuesday/Thursday lunch meetings, and then order something light off the menu.

GOAL: I will eat three healthy home-cooked dinners a week for the next three months.			
Strategy:	Action Step 1	Action Step 2	Action Step 3
Learn How to Cook	Look online and find 10 simple dinner recipes.	Sign up for a Mediterranean cooking class at my local natural food store.	Watch five episodes of "So Simple A Monkey Could Cook It" on YouTube.

Notice how even with similar healthy eating goals, your tactics can vary significantly based on your strategy. Someone who cooks will approach eating healthy dinners differently from someone who does not cook.

GOAL: I will eat a healthy dinner every night this month even when I am working late.			
Strategy:	Action Step 1	Action Step 2	Action Step 3
Plan Ahead.	Keep my fridge stocked with a few prepared healthy alternatives.	Identify one healthy restaurant that is on my way home from work.	Sign up for a healthy meal delivery service.

GOAL: I will try two new healthy gluten-free grains in the next four weeks.			
Strategy:	Action Step 1	Action Step 2	Action Step 3
Focus on Breakfast.	Read a gluten-free cookbook.	Experiment with a new gluten-free pancake recipe.	Try a new hot cereal recipe that is gluten-free.

3. **Identify any resources needed to implement your action steps.** While creating your action steps, you will find that you often need additional resources to complete them. You may already have some of the resources, such as an Internet connection to watch YouTube videos to learn something new or an alarm clock to wake up earlier to exercise. But you will likely also need to obtain additional resources that you don't already have to fulfill your action steps.

   Gather what you need. In the above examples, some resources you may need to acquire include: the cookbook you plan on reading, the healthy ingredients you plan on preparing, the cooking class you plan on taking, a lunchbox, running shoes, a probiotic, a new water bottle, and a blender for making your smoothies. Happy shopping!

   Recruit some help. Some of the resources you need may be *human* resources. Do you need to recruit additional help, such as a personal trainer, chef, or naturopath in order to accomplish your action steps? If so, check with your network of friends, family, and contacts for recommendations. Look at online reviews. Talk to people you are already working with to see if they can make a referral. When all else fails, ask that know-it-all Siri.

4. **Define your timeline.** Each action step should have an assigned due date. When do you want to have that new cookbook? When do you want to try that new recipe? Aligning every step with a date ensures that you hold yourself accountable.

You also want to make sure you associate a date with the resources you will be obtaining. If you specifically wanted your new hot tub in time for winter but you don't order it until January and it takes five weeks to arrive, you'll be stuck freezing your tatas off for a while.

Your Turn: Create an Action Plan

1. *Identify your strategy* by asking yourself "How am I going to accomplish my goal?"

2. *Create a separate mini action plan,* starting with the highest-priority goal you designed in Chapter 4 (this should be one of your one-month goals) and using the format below. Note: You may wish to use more than one strategy for the same goal. No problem. Just be sure to also create a separate mini action plan for each strategy.

MINI ACTION PLAN GOAL: <FILL IN>			
Strategy: **<Fill in>**	Action Step 1 <Fill in>	Action Step 2 <Fill in>	Action Step 3 <Fill in>
Deadline	Write in your deadline for Action Step 1.	Write in your deadline for Action Step 2	Write in your deadline for Action Step 3.
Resources Needed	List any resources needed to complete this action step.	List any resources needed to complete this action step.	List any resources needed to complete this action step.

You can download a copy of this template at **jillginsberg.com/templates.**

3. ***Make a list of the key resources needed***, then write down the details surrounding each required resource. You should identify what or who you need, when you need it, and where or how you will obtain it.

Example 1

I need a badass Ninja blender for making smoothies by next week. On Saturday I am going to buy one from Amazon Prime since that doesn't require me to leave the house. Or interact with people. Or wear a bra.

What's going in my schedule? Order blender.
When: This Saturday

Example 2

I need a lunchbox to transport my food to work. Tomorrow I'm going to go to Target to purchase one of the varieties that comes with a built-in cooler. I don't trust the fridge at my office. My co-workers would steal breast milk out of it if they were thirsty enough.

What's going in my schedule? Purchase lunchbox at Target.
When: Tomorrow

Example 3

I need to make an appointment with a naturopath who specializes in digestive health so she can recommend a good probiotic and help me figure out why I'm pooping constipated little rabbit turds. I'm going to talk to Amy about it when we meet for brunch on Sunday since I know she recently saw someone who helped her.

What's going in my schedule? Get contact info for Amy's naturopath.
When: This Sunday

4. ***Enter all relevant tasks and dates into your schedule,*** including the tasks and dates associated with acquiring additional resources or help.

5. ***Fill in your Weekly Action Plan template.*** It's not enough to create your mini action plan, enter your action steps into your planner or calendar, and then hope for the best. Take it a step further and use the template below to create a weekly action plan.

You can download a copy of this template at **jillginsberg.com/templates**. At the start of each new week print the template out, fill it in and post it somewhere highly visible!

Each week you'll want to create a new Weekly Action Plan in accordance with your current goals, strategy and action steps.

Weekly Action Plan

Current Goal		Week of		
	Action steps	Resources Needed	Completed?	Notes
Monday				
Tuesday				
Wednesday				
Thursday				
Friday				
Saturday				
Sunday				

Staying Accountable to Your Plan

Accountability is a management process that ensures the company reaches its performance goals. The first part of the equation in creating a culture of accountability is to ensure that employees have a clear understanding of the results they are expected to produce, when the result should be achieved, and how success is being measured. This is exactly what you just did when you created your SMART goals and action plan.

The second part of the accountability equation is performance reviews. In the most successful cases, employees provide frequent status updates to the management team who, in turn, regularly reports to the board of directors and shareholders.

These systems of checks and balances help ensure that duties are fulfilled and targets are met. If a business isn't meeting its objectives, management is expected to understand where they fell short and how they are going to get back on track.

Part Two of this book is going to show you how to stay accountable to your self-health as if you were running a business—because, in many respects, you are! You'll learn how to get out of your own way so you can fulfill your action steps and honor your goals. You'll also learn some special tricks for managing your time, mitigating risk, tracking your progress, and correcting your course if you fall off track.

But here are a couple of things you can start doing now as you create your action plan that will make it easier to be accountable.

Find an accountability partner. Having someone who can hold you accountable for your goals is a great source of motivation. Whether you choose a friend, a family member, or a co-worker, select someone who supports the change you are making. Communicate your action steps and timeframe, and encourage them to follow up with you on your progress. Let them tag along to the store while you stock up on all those healthy foods you can't pronounce. Perhaps they'll even agree to be your gluten-free recipe guinea pig. Refer back to your goals often. You had a specific vision in mind when you created your one-month, three-month, and six-month goals in Chapter 4. When it comes time to make your Weekly Action Plan, be sure to refer back to your most recent goals so you can keep creating compatible action steps and stay on track with your self-healthy intentions.

Schedule an appointment with yourself. My coaching clients know that every two weeks we're going to meet and I'm going to ask about their progress. It's a good idea to set a 15-minute standing (or sitting!) appointment with yourself each week so you can make sure you are making headway with your action steps. Find a consistent time each week. Then take a few minutes to assess your progress and create the next week's action plan. You can do this almost any-time—when you're riding the bus to work, after you drop the kids off at sports practice, or when you're in the bathroom hiding from the rest of your family. The key is to schedule this standing appointment at a consistent time of week so it becomes a habit.

As helpful as it is to have a coach or a management team checking in on you, you are totally capable of keeping yourself on task like a boss... as you are about to see!

PART TWO:

PROTECTING YOUR WELLIONS

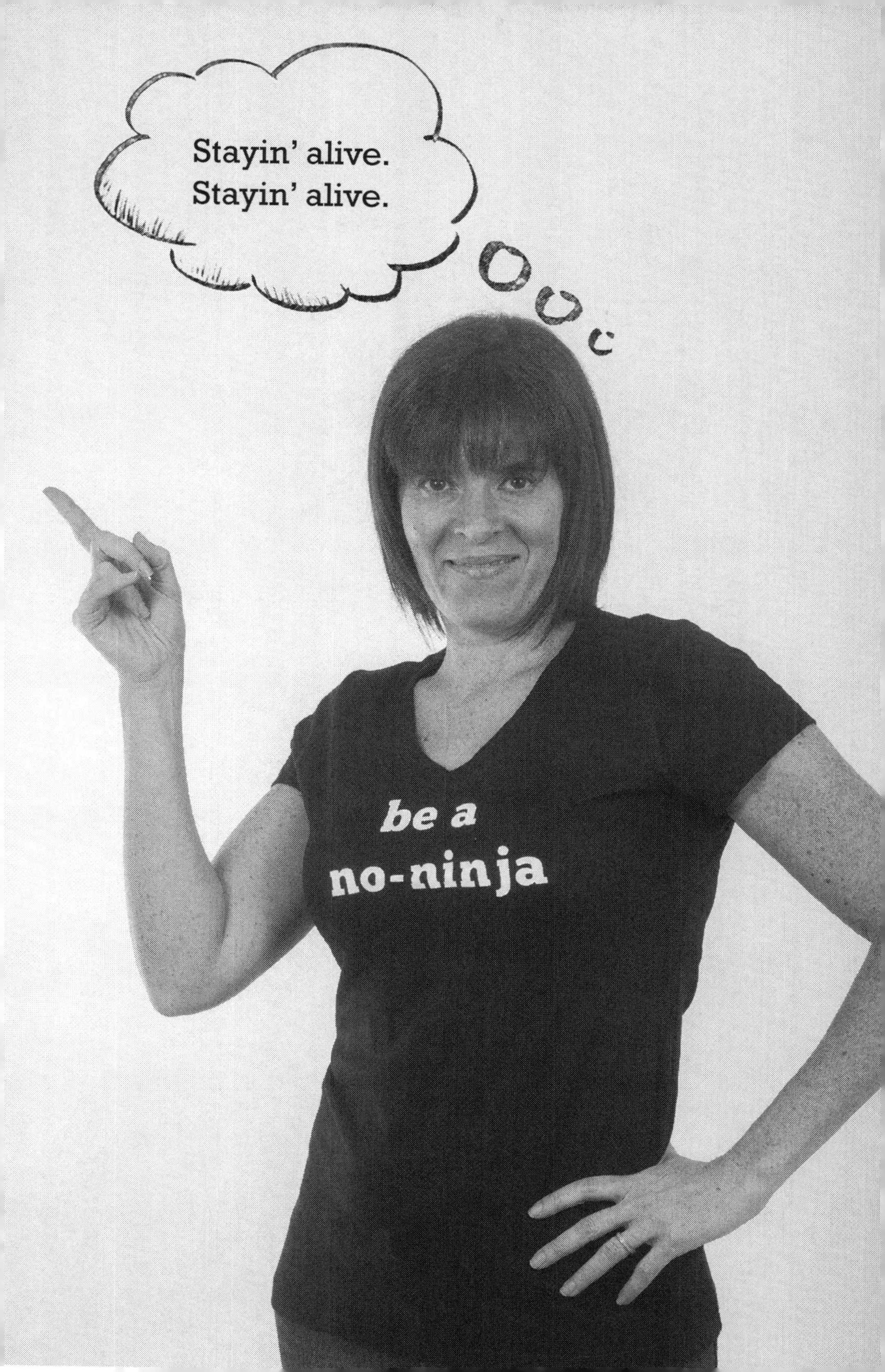
Stayin' alive.
Stayin' alive.
be a
no-ninja

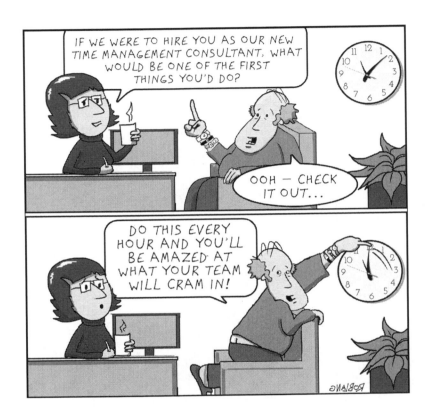

CHAPTER 6

Time Is Money, Honey: Time Management Tips

You have some exciting new goals, and you're ready to take action! Just look at you—all motivated and inspired to make self-healthy change! Nothing's getting in your way!

Such unabashed enthusiasm is great. Lots of people start off feeling exactly the same.

Take Sarah, for instance. She's totally gung-ho about doing her 30-minute strength training routine three times per week. She's off to an impressive start! Monday she does the whole workout before leaving for work. Same with Wednesday. On Friday she actually does an extra set of squats. What a proud little moment that is! She even tries to fist bump her Labradoodle, which doesn't end well. But I digress.

Then the following Monday rolls around and Sarah has to be in the office early for a monthly team meeting. So she skips the exercise routine and vows to do it when she gets home. Except on her evening commute she gets stuck in a horrendous traffic jam because some distracted, texting d-bag accidentally uses the onramp as an offramp. By the time Sarah finally makes it through her door, she has carpool tunnel syndrome and is too fried to lift a can of soup let alone a twelve-pound free weight.

Wednesday she oversleeps and only manages to get in 10 minutes of exercise. By Friday, Sarah's initial eagerness has totally waned and is replaced by such a nagging sense of guilt she is considering altogether abandoning her goal of getting in shape.

This is a common predicament. When things get hectic it's easy to use stress as an excuse not to exercise, eat healthy, or keep up with that obscure hobby you finally started working on.

The real reason why goals get derailed isn't because we oversleep, get stuck in traffic, or have busy schedules.

It's because we fail to manage our time well.

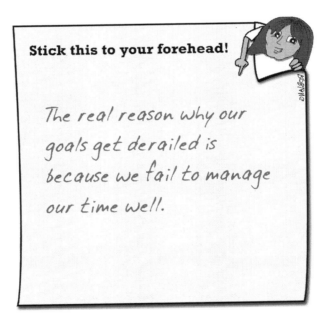

Stick this to your forehead!

The real reason why our goals get derailed is because we fail to manage our time well.

Time Is Your Limiting Factor

In business, a "limiting factor" is a variable that restricts or limits production or sale of a given product. These are the circumstances that hold a business back and distract it from being successful or reaching its goals. Common limiting factors for businesses include financial constraints, manufacturing capacity, inadequate staffing, or immature technology.

When it comes to being a Wellionaire, there are also limiting factors that impact productivity, such as money and physical capability. But time tends to be the most common limiting factor that can keep you from reaching your goals. Regardless of how motivated or enthusiastic you are about making self-healthy change, there are only so many hours in a day. So it's essential that you learn how to use them well.

Stick this to your forehead!

From Google to a multitude of apps, there are lots of calendar tools available. But the best one I've found—and the tool I personally use—is a physical planner called The Freedom Planner. Part calendar, part goal journal and part motivational notebook, it will change the way you approach each week. Another alternative is The Passion Planner.

Time Management Tips

Now that you have clearly defined your action steps, you want to make sure nothing gets in the way of fulfilling them. One of the best ways to mitigate the risk of abandoning your self-healthy goals is to reclaim your time. Here are six strategies for effective time management.

1. **Look ahead.** Looking ahead allows you to process what's about to happen so you can understand the impact your scheduled activities will have on your wellness goals before they derail you. If you look

several days to a week ahead in your calendar, it makes it easy to spot potential wellthcare roadblocks and adjust accordingly.

For instance, you may notice that you're traveling for half the week to a location that doesn't have a gym. Hell, they barely have indoor plumbing. So you switch up your schedule and squeeze in a couple of extra workouts before leaving town. Not only do you succeed in hitting your exercise goals for the week, you even remember to pack your exercise band so you can do some strength training on the road.

Or you might notice that you have to work later one evening, leaving you less time to cook a healthy meal for your family. Knowing that you are going to be extra busy in advance allows you to plan accordingly. Pulled BBQ crockpot chicken to the rescue! Better yet, add a splash of bourbon when you get home after the kids have eaten.

2. **Chunk your time**. One of the best ways to improve your productivity and efficiency is to group related action items together in batches. For example, on Sunday evening you can slice and dice your veggies for the entire week. This will save you meal prep time later. Or try running all your errands on Saturday instead of one at a time throughout the week. Group your housework together. Pull on a pair of rubber gloves and knock it all out in one dreaded session. You can even schedule all your phone calls for the same afternoon if possible, including the one you've been putting off for weeks to your under-medicated sister-in-law.

By clustering similar activities, you create more room in your schedule for other activities that inspire or benefit you.

3. **Outsource activities.** Yeah, we get it. You're Superwoman. You can check homework, chew gum, and wipe someone else's butt all at the same time. While standing on one leg. Texting. In heels!

Clearly you're skilled, talented, gifted, and competent. But you're still not capable of doing everything yourself. At least not doing it well.

Nobody is. And no business is either. That's why they routinely out-source activities such as accounting, manufacturing, and customer support to entities that can do the job better and more efficiently. The company then gets to focus on developing its core competencies—the unique functions it performs best.

Just like every business has limited resources, so do you. That's why you need to quit sinking your resources into the stuff you're not good at! Your weakness is another person's strength, so focus on what you know and outsource what you don't. Redistributing some of your work will free up your time and increase your capacity to get other things done. Then you can focus more on what really matters. Like being a Wellionaire! Or crocheting your dog a tail warmer.

- **_Hire other people._** Farm out the stuff you hate doing or are terrible at doing, and focus on what you do best. Stressed out by shopping for recipes with more than four ingredients? No biggie. Use a delivery service like Blue Apron. Can't cook a pot of rice to save your ass(et) and not interested in learning how? That's what Munchery is for! Does the thought of cleaning a toilet activate your gag reflex? Hand the scrubber over to Merry Maids! They actually enjoy cleaning toilets. Why do you think they're so merry in the first place? If going to Costco makes your third eye twitch, get someone from Task Rabbit to fill up that freakishly large, ankle biter of a grocery cart for you.
- **_Do a quick cost-benefit analysis._** Before you start complaining about how there's no extra money to pay for help, do a quick cost-benefit analysis. It's an analytical tool businesses use to assess the pros and cons of moving forward with an idea or proposal. In other words, you want to determine the benefit of paying someone to clean your house versus the cost of going fucking insane. You do the math.

4. **Delegate.** Not everyone's made of money! But you don't have to rely on paid services to help increase your capacity. Look around and you'll see there's plenty of free help to be found. I mean, isn't that what teenagers are for? And isn't your mother getting bored in retirement? You know she's just dying to sew that Halloween costume!

Make use of the resources already at your disposal by delegating some of the tasks you don't want to or can't do yourself:

- **Trade tasks.** For instance, maybe you're yearning for some kid-free peace and quiet and have a friend who just loves kids. She, on the other hand, happens to hate anything related to cooking. Boy is she kicking herself for signing up to make 70 dozen cookies for tomorrow's school bake sale. Why not trade? You take her 40 pounds of baking supplies while she watches your four small children. Just don't forget that you actually have to take them back. Yes. All four of them.
- **Put your kids to work.** Speaking of children, if they could toil in the fields back in the 1800s and early 1900s then, damn it, it's okay to ask them to fold a freaking load of laundry every now and then. Little people are quite capable, and those tiny, adorable hands are useful for more than just fitting into small spaces. Put them to work and give yourself a break. There are lots of chores they can help with, from dish washing to bed making to weeding—otherwise known as the modern day version of agrarian labor.

5. **Team up to get it done.** Call it a joint venture. Call it an alliance. Call it whatever you want. Just find others who have the same needs as you. Pool your resources and divvy up the expense and the workload. Join a nanny share so you don't have to pay for childcare all on your own. Find a preschool co-op where you can volunteer for a couple of hours in exchange for some childcare. Sign up for a cooking club where each week you prepare one meal and receive ten different meals that taste much better in return. There are all sorts of creative ways to free up some of your time and save your sanity.

6. **Defend your time.** This is the hardest one for us overachievers. I know people who put fake meetings in their work calendar to protect themselves from the all-too-famous Outlook over-schedulers. And you know what? It's brilliant! There's nothing worse than sitting around in a conference room all day, bored out of your mind, dopey-eyed and drooling, listening to people go on and on about nonsense when you could be getting actual real work done. When it comes to defending your time, you have to be aggressive:

- **Be a No Ninja.** Don't take on more than you can handle. Say yes to the opportunities that are in line with your vision. But say "no thanks" to the tasks, projects, and drama that people can deal with themselves or that aren't in line with your priorities and goals.
- **For heaven's sake get off the damn Internet.** Facebook? Twitter? Instagram? Incessant Inbox checking? Stop wasting time in the tech void and slowly step away from your electronics before you become a full-fledged mouse potato. Turn off your social media notifications. Stop taking pictures of your lunch. Silence your phone. Set limits on your screen time just like you would for your children. Make the beeping, buzzing, and ringing stop and you'll be amazed at what you can start doing.
- **Block out your schedule.** You should have already done this in Chapter 5, but, if you haven't already, remember to schedule your key action steps. By putting these tasks on your calendar, you are protecting that time and making your action steps a priority. Remember: It never hurts to schedule a fake meeting or two, especially if you work in an office. Even an over-scheduler won't dare mess with your standing Friday afternoon gynecologist appointment.

How to Find More Time in Your Schedule for Wellthcare

Now that you know how to stop wasting so much time, you can dedicate your reclaimed time toward getting self-healthy.

Follow these five simple steps:

1. **Record how you spend your time.** Before you can begin to manage your time, the first thing you need to do is get a clear picture of how you're spending it. Putting your daily activities down on paper is the first step toward making room for the things in life that really matter.

2. **Evaluate your schedule to figure out what's wasting your time or energy.** There are lots of "time thieves" in our lives. Look at how you spend your time and observe where you're losing minutes, hours, or even days. Three frequent time- and energy-wasting culprits include the Internet, television, and, last but not least, tiresome humans (particularly of the overly dramatic or self-absorbed variety).

3. **Stop doing those things!** Cut back on these draining behaviors or stop engaging with them altogether and you'll preserve your energy and create space for more important activities.

4. **Notice where there are gaps of time where you can fit in healthier habits.** Once you ditch those time wasters, you'll see that there's really plenty of room left for nutrition, exercise, and other forms of self-care.

5. **Create a Self-Healthy Living Schedule.** This is a weekly planning tool I created to help my clients keep their ducks in a row. It combines the regular day-to-day activities you have to do, such as work and family obligations, with the activities you want to do to stay healthy, such as preparing nutritious meals, working out, and taking care of yourself. It even leaves room for aspirational activities you only wish you had time to do. You'll find a template on page 69.

Your Turn: Manage YOUR Time

1) Complete a "Day in the Life" Exercise

You can download a copy of this template at **jillginsberg.com/templates.**

Starting from when you wake up in the morning until bedtime, write down how you spend a typical WEEKDAY in your life. Note the approximate time when you complete each task. (If you don't have a "typical" day, I recommend completing this exercise several days in a row so you can spot patterns.)

Be real with yourself about how you spend your time. Include things like "Playing FarmVille" for three hours and "Uploading food porn to Instagram" for 90 minutes. It may not be pretty, but it's the truth.

While you want to include a lot of details, there's no need to include everything. Some things are better left in the bathroom. Or the bedroom. Or even a padded room. (Freak.)

Weekday Example:

- 5:30 a.m., Wake up
- 5:45 a.m., Think about showering
- 6:15 a.m., Eat Breakfast
- 6:30 a.m., Leave for Work

TIME: TASK:

1. _____
2. _____
3. _____
4. _____
5. _____
6. _____
7. _____
8. _____
9. _____
10. _____
11. _____
12. _____
13. _____
14. _____
15. _____

Now write down how you spend a typical WEEKEND in your life. It's likely quite different from how you spend your weekdays.

Weekend Example:

- Saturday, 10 a.m., Meet Amy for our Saturday morning stair climb
- Saturday, 1 p.m., Get walked by my dogs
- Saturday 7 p.m., Date night
- Sunday 9 a.m., Confess my date night sins in church
- Sunday 11 a.m., Brunch
- Sunday 3 p.m., Grocery shopping and errands

TIME: TASK:

1. _____
2. _____
3. _____
4. _____
5. _____
6. _____
7. _____
8. _____
9. _____
10. _____
11. _____
12. _____
13. _____
14. _____
15. _____

Take a few minutes to review your completed "Day in the Life" exercise before moving on to the next step. Look closely at how you spend your time. You may be noticing blocks of inefficiencies. If you are like most people, you're probably spending at least an hour a day on unproductive tasks that could be put on hold or completely eliminated from your schedule. Which leads us to the next step...

2) Complete the Time Management Exercise

You can download a copy of this worksheet at **jillginsberg.com/ templates.**

This exercise will help you figure out what's draining you and what you wish you could be doing instead. Refer back to the answers you provided in the "Day in the Life" exercise. Be brutally honest about what you don't like doing, what you need help doing, or what you could stop doing altogether.

Top three things I'm doing that I actually enjoy doing:
1. _____
2. _____

3. _____

Examples: Walking my kids to school each morning; yoga class; my new job

Top three things I'm doing that I don't like/dread/hate doing:
1. _____
2. _____
3. _____

Examples: Cleaning my house; paying the monthly bills; helping the kids with homework

Top three areas where I can be more efficient:
1. _____
2. _____
3. _____

Examples: Sorting/washing/folding laundry; checking emails; my morning routine

The area I most need to be more efficient in is

_____

Example: My morning routine.

Top 3 things I can do to save time in this area:
1. _____
2. _____
3. _____

Examples: Make lunches the night before; lay out my clothes the night before; stop hitting the snooze button 14 times

Which activities seem to drain you?
1. _____
2. _____
3. _____

Examples: Phone conversations with "that" friend; watching television; driving to and from work

The activity I most want to do less of is _____.
Example: Driving to and from work

The activity I most want to get help with is _____.
Example: Paying the monthly bills

The activity I most want to stop doing altogether is _____.
Example: Cleaning the house

What do you wish you could be doing more of?

1. _____
2. _____
3. _____

Examples: Spending time with my family; traveling; reading

The activity I most want to do more of is:_____.
Example: Spending time with my family

Things I would try doing if I had more time:

1. _____
2. _____
3. _____

Examples: Blogging; scuba diving; learning Spanish

The activity I would most want to try if I had more time is:

_____.

Example: Scuba diving

3) Make Room in Your Schedule

Pay special attention to your responses regarding what you wish you could do less of, get help with, or stop doing altogether. These are your time thieves and they are not only draining your time, they're depleting precious energy.

You want to model yourself after the concept of "lean manufacturing." When companies practice lean manufacturing, they eliminate as much waste as possible from the manufacturing process. That's exactly what you're trying to do with your day-to-day schedule.

Steal some hours back by finding smarter ways to complete your daily activities. Be more productive. Outsource. Delegate. Team up. The best way to find more time is to minimize wasted time.

1. *Decide how you are going to delegate/outsource/team up to complete this activity:*

The activity I most want to do less of is _____ .

I'm going to accomplish this by _____ .

Example 1:
The activity I most want to do less of is driving to and from work. I'm going to accomplish this by taking the bus.

Example 2:
The activity I most want to do less of is cleaning up the shitstorm that is my kitchen after dinner. I'm going to accomplish this by delegating this task to the kids. Right after I remove all sharp objects that could be used to stab someone.

2. *Decide how you are going to delegate/outsource/team up to complete this activity:*

The activity I most want to get help with is _____ .

I'm going to I am going to accomplish this by _____ .

Example 1:
The activity I most want to get help with is paying the bills. I'm going to accomplish this by asking my husband if he can take on this task since I've been doing it for the past ten years. It's his turn.

Example 2:
The activity I most want to get help with is babysitting. I'm going to accomplish this by signing up for the local babysitting co-op. Here's to hoping all the good kids show up when it's my turn. #prayforme #needamiracle

3. *Decide how you are going to delegate/outsource/team up to complete this activity:*

The activity I most want to stop doing altogether is _____ .

I'm going to accomplish this by _____ .

Example 1:
The activity I most want to stop doing altogether is cleaning the house. I'm going to accomplish this by hiring someone to do a deep cleaning twice a month.

Example 2:
The activity I most want to stop doing altogether is mowing the lawn. I'm going to accomplish this by hiring my neighbor's teenager to do the job. I have so much dirt on that kid, how could he possibly say no to eight cents an hour?

4. *Decide how you can do this activity more efficiently:*

The area I most need to be more efficient in is _____ .

I can be more efficient in this area by _____ .

Example 1:
The area I most need to be more efficient in is my morning routine. I can be more efficient in this area by making lunches and laying out my clothes the night before.

Example 2:
The area I most need to be more efficient in is dinner preparation. I can be more efficient in this area by creating a meal plan in advance.

4) Create a Self-Healthy Living Schedule

Now that you've figured out how to be more efficient with your time and created some room in your schedule, you can create your own Self-Healthy Living Schedule. Instructions are on page 70.

Sample Self-Healthy Living Schedule	M	T	W	Th	F	Sat	Sun
				TIME			
EVERYDAY ACTIVITIES:							
Wake up							
Get Ready							
Arrive at Work							
Eat Breakfast							
Lunch							
Healthy Snack							
Leave Work							
Arrive Home							
Eat Dinner/Clean up/Make lunch for next day							
Read/Write/TV Bed							
OTHER WEEKLY TASKS							
Meal Planning							
Grocery Shopping							
Weekly Errands							
SOCIAL ACTIVITIES							
Date Night							
Fun Night							
Social Time with Friends							
EXERCISE							
Gym/Fitness Class/Other Exercise							
SPIRITUALITY, GROWTH, SELF-CARE							
Weekly Self Care Time/Misc Appointments/Hobbies							

You can download a copy of this template at **jillginsberg.com/templates.**

The difference between your Self-Healthy Living Schedule and your Wellness Acton Plan is that your Wellness Action Plan can change frequently. Your Self-Healthy Living Schedule should stay fairly constant, with the exception of big life transitions and seasonal schedule changes.

- Start by including your work, family, and basic personal/hygiene obligations under the "Everyday Activities" section.
- In the "Other Weekly Tasks" section insert those healthy lifestyle tasks that you can cluster into once-a-week occurrences, such as errands, meal planning, and grocery shopping.
- Under "Social Activities" add in the events that keep you connected to your loved ones, such as date night, family outings, and time with friends.
- Under "Exercise" schedule in all the forms of fitness you currently do or will be doing to meet your goals.
- Add in at least one self-care activity or hobby in the "Spirituality, Growth, and Self-Care" section, such as a massage, pedicure, class, wine guzzling, or other soul-fulfilling endeavor (who says wine guzzling isn't soul-fulfilling?).

It's up to you to follow through with the commitments you just outlined above. Organize your resources and take charge of your time so you can stay on track with your goals and action steps. That's what great managers do!

Don't forget to circulate the agenda! Share your Self-Healthy Living Schedule with your accountability partner so they can check in with you, and make sure the people in your household also know your schedule so everyone can be on the same page.

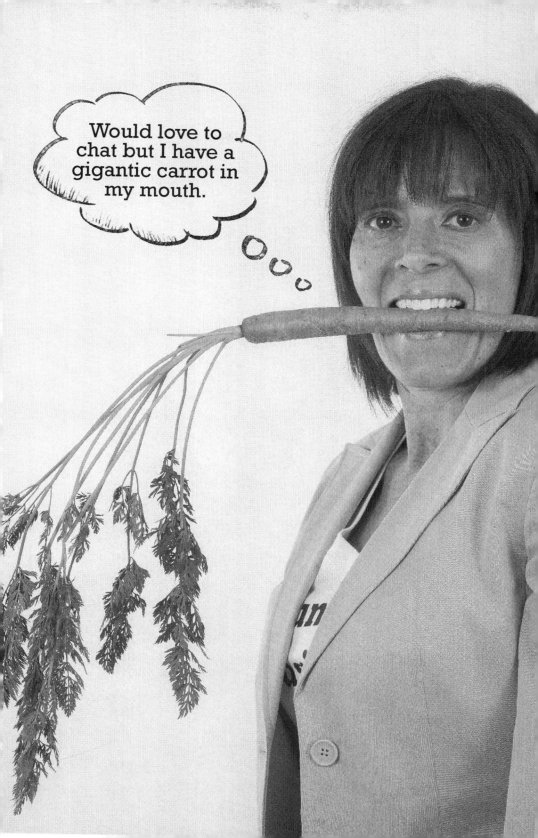

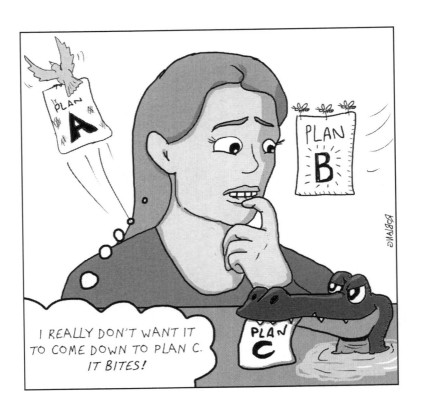

CHAPTER 7

Best-Laid Plans: Mitigating Risk

Successful managers don't just think about their current move.

They understand that unforeseen events occur, so they think several steps ahead, anticipate outcomes, and make contingency plans. This is precisely what you need to do to stay on top of your wellions.

No matter how effective you are at managing your time or how determined you are to achieve your goals, things won't always go according to plan. You will eventually slip up because slip-ups are normal!

Although it's nice to be optimistic about reaching your wellness goals, you also want to be realistic. That means being prepared for little hiccups and unexpected events. In the business world, we call this risk management. It's the process of identifying possible risks and consequences, developing solutions, and implementing contingency plans. When properly implemented, a risk management plan helps ensure you accomplish your goals despite the uncertainties you may face.

What Is a Contingency Plan?
A contingency plan is your Plan B. When Plan A fails, a contingency plan helps you avoid setbacks and keeps you on track.

Plan A can go south for a number of reasons. Conditions may change. Your environment might become less predictable. Or some last-minute glitch could occur. Your contingency plan allows for an alternate path toward achieving your goals should your original plans fall apart. It is not, however, an excuse to act like a fool.

The Wrong Way to Manage Risk

Say, for example, you happen to be lactose intolerant. When you eat dairy your insides feel like a Category 5 storm surge. Ever since you heard your orthorexic cousin refer to cheese as "cow pus" you hardly ever crave it anymore, though you still have a bit of a weakness/obsession/borderline fetish for soft cheeses. So, generally, you take pains to avoid rendezvousing with said soft cheeses. When you have an unexpected run-in with some baked brie at your best friend's cocktail party, in a momentary lapse of self-control, you completely fondle your face with it. Having succumbed to its ooey-gooey seduction, you now have to resort to Plan B. This entails you downing a couple of Lactaid and thanking "the big guy in the sky" that your girlfriend happens to be out of town so you can spare her the torment of having to share a bed with your intestines. As far as back-up plans go, this one isn't going to win first prize. Popping a Lactaid is more of a Band-Aid solution than a contingency plan. Well thought out contingency plans aren't reactionary. Instead they take a more preemptive approach.

The Right Way to Manage Risk

One of the most effective ways to mitigate risk is to anticipate setbacks and notice red flags. This is especially important when it comes to managing common Wellionaire risks, because a shame spiral can come into play after slip-ups.

The best way to preemptively avoid common risks isn't to anticipate and have a plan in place for dealing with slip-ups. It's to anticipate and have a plan in place for avoiding slip-ups whenever possible.

In other words, take steps to reduce the likelihood that the risk will occur in the first place. Instead of taking a Lactaid after the fact, you could instead ask your best friend to preemptively stab you in the hand with a dull knife if he sees you even so much as make eye contact with the baked brie. Or better yet, eat a dairy-free, creamy snack before you go to the party to help quench your lust.

Again, you won't always be able to get it perfect. But if you can prevent setbacks most of the time, you'll be in tip-top shape.

Common Wellionaire Risks

In my practice, I've found that the wellness categories most susceptible to slip-ups are related to diet management and fitness.

For example, birthdays and holiday parties are notorious for derailing even the best-laid weight-loss plans. There's something about annual traditions, buttercream frosting, and passed hors d'oeuvres that makes us go weak in the knees.

Most of us know this about ourselves. We understand that we can't rely on pure willpower to win the battle of the buttercream. If your intention is not to eat the icing, heading into a birthday party without a back-up plan is pretty much the same thing as giving in to the temptation. Because, more than likely, you'll start by dipping your fingertip into someone else's icing only to end up licking your own plate. Twice.

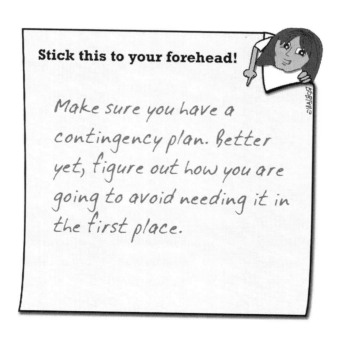

Stick this to your forehead!

Make sure you have a contingency plan. Better yet, figure out how you are going to avoid needing it in the first place.

So if your goal is to lose 12 pounds in 12 weeks, and you have a string of family birthdays coming up, you're probably going to struggle to meet your weight loss goals.

Unless, of course, you create a risk management plan to help see you through.

Types of Risk Management Strategies

When protecting your wellions, there are three risk management strategies that are helpful to consider:

1. ***Hedging—The act of making a balancing or compensating transaction to protect yourself against making the wrong choice.***
You've probably heard the familiar phrase "hedging your bets" to refer to situations in which one tries to increase their financial chances of success. A non-financial example of hedging is to pack your cycling shoes and running shoes in your gym bag the night before. If you don't wake up in time to join the rest of the nutjobs at the 5:30 a.m. spin class, you can at least jump on the treadmill for 30 minutes and still get in a decent workout. By packing both sets of shoes, you're protecting yourself against failing to meet your exercise goals.

2. ***Taking Out an "Insurance Policy"—The act of creating a back-up plan to protect yourself against failure.***
Using the same fitness scenario, an example of taking out an insurance policy is to block out some time on your calendar in the evening to ride the recumbent bike that typically collects dust in your garage. It's not your first choice. But if your spin class doesn't happen, it will do in a pinch, and at least you'll sleep better knowing you managed to squeeze in your workout. If you end up exercising as originally planned in the morning—bonus!—you'll have some free time to finally shave your legs. Or trim your nose hairs. Or both.

Another example of having "insurance" is to make sure you always have healthy frozen foods on hand in case your plans change and you don't have time to cook dinner. Stocking your freezer with convenient nutritious foods such as frozen fish filets, chicken breasts, or shelled edamame is essentially an insurance policy against ordering takeout or eating 10-day-old mystery leftovers.

3. ***Setting Controls—Creating systems to make sure you stay within the boundaries you set for yourself.***

   Continuing with our fitness theme, an example of setting controls is to pre-register for spin class. Plunking down real money on a non-refundable class is a great way to make sure you don't sleep through that alarm. Or try using a tool like HassleMe. Just decide how often you want to be reminded about a goal, and the app will send reminders to your inbox. Enter when you want to be hassled and type the exact message you want to appear. For instance: "Don't forget to make sweet love to that bike saddle three times this week!"

   Another example of setting controls is not purchasing a temptation food. If you know that you turn into a rabid animal anytime you get in the same room with a bag of potato chips, and you're looking to cut back on eating junk food, don't buy the potato chips in the first place. If it's not in your home, you're far less likely to end up in a staring contest with the bottom of the bag. You can either try substituting a less fattening version of potato chips, such as Pop Chips, or—better still—eliminate the salty craving altogether. Setting controls around which foods you keep in your home is a cravings management tool.

These strategies can help protect you against slip-ups and are the basis of any wellness-related risk management plan.

How to Create a Risk Management Plan

There are three simple steps to creating an effective risk management plan:

1. ***Identify the risks.*** The first step is to perform a basic risk assessment. This means determining which aspects of your wellness plan may be most susceptible to slip-ups. Warning: This part can be a little anxiety inducing because you are basically imagining yourself failing. But it's important to keep things in perspective and understand that the whole point of this exercise is to avoid failing in the first place.

   For each objective, go ahead and anticipate the potential challenges. Think about the circumstances and situations that might make your action steps difficult to fulfill. Hint: Look back at the "Threat" section of your SWOT analysis. The concerns you outlined should definitely be considered risks.

When thinking about other possible risks, you want to think about external factors, such as your environment, and internal factors, such as your attitude. Create a list of all challenges that come to mind. Then quickly move on to the next step before your anxiety turns into a full-fledged panic attack.

Examples of Wellionaire risks include:
- You recently discovered you have a sensitivity to gluten. Tonight you are invited to your Italian neighbor's house for dinner. When you were out watering your plants this morning you saw her polishing her stainless steel pasta maker.
- You are committed to exercising 30 minutes every day to help reduce your cholesterol. Except you are about to leave on an RV adventure and will mostly be holed up in a 25-foot house on wheels, tearin' up the slow lane, for the next two weeks straight.
- You intend to lose one pound per week but your mom is visiting from out of town for an entire week. Her greatest joy in life is stuffing you full of her homemade desserts, especially those famous cream puffs. She loads up her car with butter, heavy cream, and powdered sugar.

2. **Estimate the impact of the risk.** In order to know how to alleviate the risk, you need to know what the potential impact is. Ask yourself "How will this risk impact my goals?"

   Examples of estimating the impact of risk include:
   - Situation: Dinner at the neighbor's house when you have a sensitivity to gluten.
     Impact of the risk: Eating gluten and feeling sick afterward.
   - Situation: RV adventure threatens to derail your 30-minutes-per-day exercise plan.
     Impact of the risk: Not exercising and negatively impacting your cholesterol levels.
   - Situation: Mom's visiting and plans to bake decadent sweet treats all week long.
     Impact of the risk: Not losing weight. Hell, let's be real. You're worried you're going to gain back all the weight you've lost so far.

3. **Reduce/eliminate the risk.** Next you want to brainstorm ways to overcome each challenge identified in Step 1 so you can mitigate the risk. Ask yourself "What can be done to reduce the likelihood of this risk?" and "What can be done to manage the risk, should it occur?"

Remember to consider the risk management strategies that were outlined earlier in the chapter. Think about how you can hedge, provide some insurance, or implement a control mechanism to help reduce or eliminate the likelihood of failure.

For instance, if you're concerned that you may compromise your weight-loss goal by continuing to overeat at dinner, possible controls include waiting 20 minutes before helping yourself to another serving, using a smaller plate, putting your fork down between bites, or chewing each bite 30 times (thereby causing everyone else at the table to go into a fit of apoplectic rage). If you're out to dinner, you could also hedge by splitting a meal with a health-conscious friend and letting him or her decide what to order. Hope you like kelp noodles! Or you could provide yourself with some insurance by asking the waiter to only bring out half your meal and request that he pack up the other half to go.

Other examples of how to mitigate wellth risk include:
- Situation: Dinner at the neighbor's house when you have a sensitivity to gluten.
  Impact of the risk: Eating gluten and feeling sick after.
  Mitigation Suggestions—Insurance: Offer to bring a gluten-free dish to dinner so you know you will have something to eat. Hedge: Eat a light snack before dinner so you don't come to the table starving. This will make it less likely that you will end up eating the pasta.
- Situation: RV adventure threatens to derail your 30-minutes-per-day exercise plan.
  Impact of the risk: Not exercising and negatively impacting your cholesterol levels.
  Mitigation Suggestions—Insurance: Download a "bodyweight exercise routine" that you can do anywhere or go for a walk every evening of the trip, walking 15 minutes away from wherever you're parked before turning around.

Control: Make a pact with your family that you won't eat any s'mores until you've gotten your 30 minutes of exercise in. That should be pretty motivating considering the opportunity to stuff yourself with s'mores every day is the whole reason you agreed to go on the trip in the first place.

- Situation: Mom's visiting and plans to bake decadent sweet treats all week long.
  Impact of the risk: Not losing weight or possibly even gaining weight.
  Mitigation Suggestions— Control: Tell mom the oven is broken and, sadly, isn't being serviced until the day after she leaves. Hedge: Double your servings of fruits and veggies to make sure you fill up on the good stuff. Then there won't be much room left for mom's goodies.

Other Important Considerations for Risk Management

Here are some other key points to remember as you implement your risk management plan:

- **Communicate with your peeps.** Explain to the people who are closest to you what the risks are in reaching your goals. People who love and care for you want you to succeed. If you take the time to explain the potential risk to your success, they will root for you, not sabotage you (or they're just mean). Your neighbor will be on board with you not eating her pasta if she knows you'll then be spending the rest of the evening fouling her bathroom. Mom will understand that you aren't able to enter the annual family cream-puff eating contest. Even if she thinks you're a total wuss for sitting it out. Don't be afraid to tell people what you need!
- **Continue to reevaluate the risk.** Risk management is a continuous process, not a one-time deal. After you create your plan, you want to evaluate the results of your mitigation strategies to determine their effectiveness, and revise them as needed:

- After a short period of time, check in with yourself to see how things are going. If your risk management strategy is humming along, terrific. If not, try another strategy.
- Think about what's working and which types of situations you tend to struggle with. Learn from this as you move forward with future Wellionaire goals and action steps. Be on the lookout for new risks. If you find that another obstacle is posing a threat to your success, add it to your risk management plan.

- **Ditch the all-or-nothing mentality.** When you suffer a setback or miss a target, it's tempting to give up. Don't fall into the trap of believing that if you can't execute your goals perfectly they aren't worth striving for at all. As long as you are following along with the exercises in this book, you should have a set of SMART goals that are attainable and achievable.

Even so, things won't always go according to plan despite your risk management strategies. That's the nature of life! Instead of beating yourself up for the one thing you didn't get right, focus on all the great strides you've made so far. Expect the occasional slip-up and skip the self-blame. It's not productive. Then recommit to your goals, trust that can do better tomorrow, and immediately take positive steps forward the very next day.

Your Turn: Create A Risk Management Plan

In the sample plans, I provided examples of all three risk management strategies for demonstration purposes. You don't have to do all three. Just pick the strategy or strategies that make sense for your situation.

SAMPLE 1

Plan Features	Description
Risk Factors	I have an addiction to buttercream frosting
Risks	Four family birthday parties this month = four tempting cakes
Risk Impact	1. Failing to meet my weight-loss goal 2. Increasing my sugar cravings
Strategies to Mitigate Risk	**HEDGE:** I normally allow myself two small desserts per week as part of my eating plan. Otherwise I get hangry. But I'm going to skip desserts on the weeks when there is a birthday party in case that buttercream frosting gets the best of me. **INSURANCE:** I'm going to whip up a batch of my famous black bean brownies. Trust me, they're ahhhh-mazing. I'll bring a brownie with me to each party so I have a better option if I feel like I need something sweet. **CONTROLS:** To avoid binging at any of the parties, I'm going to allow myself to have a small sliver. Between all four parties it will equal one normal-sized piece of cake.

SAMPLE 2

Plan Features	Description
Risk Factors	I don't always feel like jogging even though I set a goal of running 2 miles at the local high school track three mornings per week
Risks	-The weather. It's been super cold and/or rainy. And I live in Seattle! -My work schedule -Sore muscles
Risk Impact	1. Failing to meet my fitness goal 2. Compromising my overall health since it's rainy half the year
Strategies to Mitigate Risk	**HEDGE:** I'm taking a Pliates class at my local community center. It also meets twice per week so at least I'll have that in case I don't feel like running. (Is it really true that the core contractions are worse than labor?) **INSURANCE:** I signed up for a gym membership that I plan on keeping through the rainy months. This way I always have a place to run even when the weather sucks. **CONTROLS:** My friend Amy is going to jog with me. Knowing that she is counting on me will keep me from bailing. (Unless there's hail. I draw the line when frozen balls of precipitation start falling from the sky.)

The Bottom Line?

Companies create risk management plans to minimize setbacks and to help the business recover quickly if an obstacle occurs.

Likewise, a risk management plan improves your chances of meeting your goals and following through on your action steps. By anticipating slip-ups and creating a menu of flexible behavioral options, you will be able to adjust to whatever comes your way and stay on track!

You can download a copy of this template at **jillginsberg.com/ templates.**

Plan Features	Description
Risk Factors	
Risks	
Risk Impact	
Strategies to Mitigate Risk	**HEDGE:** **INSURANCE:** **CONTROLS:**

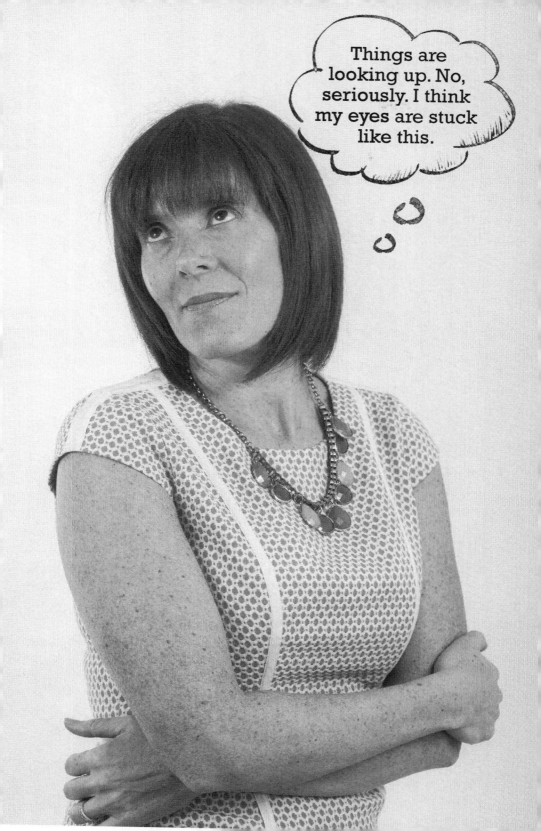

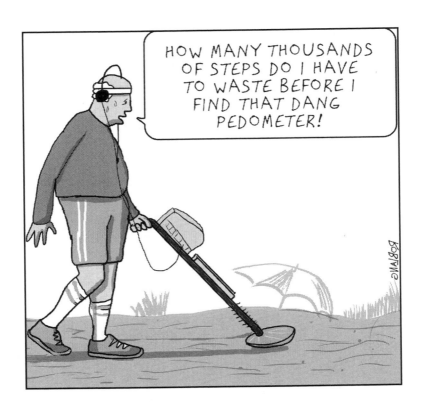

CHAPTER 8

Your Personal Balance Sheet: Tracking Your Performance

Companies use tracking tools to hold their employees accountable and to gauge whether their business objectives are being met.

Income statements, cash flow statements, balance sheets, budgets, and employee performance reviews are some of the most critical accountability tools a company has.

Likewise, you want to have a mechanism in place for keeping yourself accountable and monitoring progress toward becoming a Self-Made Wellionaire. The tracking tool you use doesn't have to be as complex as the ones used by a Fortune 500 company. In fact, it should be super easy to use! Measuring your performance consistently with a simple and reliable tracking tool will allow you to see where you are succeeding and where you are struggling.

The Importance of Tracking

Tracking tools allow businesses to measure their performance against their goals so they can clearly see where they came close to, fell short of, or exceeded expectations.

Similarly, tracking your wellness progress helps you to assess:

- How close you came to achieving your goals
- What adjustments, if any, need to be made to your goals
- What changes can be applied to improve the likelihood of hitting your goals

Before you can track your progress, though, you need to know what you are measuring in the first place.

Wellthcare Metrics

The mighty dollar may be the king metric in the business world, but it's certainly not the way to measure true wellth. Some of the more popular self-health metrics include calories, pounds, inches, and minutes—depending on the goals—although there are many other health metrics that can work just as well. You might want to lower your cholesterol score, train for a half-marathon by running a certain number of miles per day, or track your number of attempts per week toward trickier yoga poses like crow, headstand, or wheel. (Perhaps a helmet is in order if you would like to make it past attempt number one.)

You might recall that when you designed your SMART goals in Chapter 4, one of the things you had to consider was how to make your goals measurable. Let's take a look at some of the sample goals provided and identify the wellthcare metrics being used:

Goal	Metric
I will learn how to cook **one new healthy meal** per week for the next three months.	Number of meals
80% of the groceries I purchase each week will consist of fruits, veggies, and other whole foods.	Percent of groceries
I will lose **12 pounds** in 12 weeks.	Pounds
I will add **30 minutes of movement** to each weekday for three months.	Minutes

The metrics you established when you created your goals are the same metrics you will track. Your metric is always going to be associated with a number, so if you keep that in mind it should make it easier to identify.

Helpful Self-Health Tracking Tools

The key to making sure you succeed with your one-month, three-month, and six-month self-healthy goals is to track your daily performance. Tracking tools are a great way to monitor your wellness activities on a day-to-day basis so that you can meet your longer-term goals. From blood tests to body measurements to glucose meters, there are multiple ways to track just about any wellness metric.

- **Fitness apps/activity trackers.** It seems like there's a fitness app or activity tracker for every exercise, ability level, and goal you could possibly have. From running to cycling to cross training—and probably even finger wrestling, for all I know!—if you're interested in tracking it, there's an app or device that can do it. The Fitbit is a popular option but it's definitely not the only game in town. Google "fitness apps" or "activity trackers" to find lots of other viable possibilities.
- **Food journaling.** Whether you are looking to lose weight, change your eating lifestyle, or eliminate a food group from your diet, one of the keys to your success is being able to visualize patterns and identify trouble spots. Food journaling gives you a window into your eating habits and allows you to see the impact of your choices.

Although there are many ways to food journal, I've found that the simpler the tool, the more likely people are to stick with it.

You can find tons of complex online journals and apps that provide calorie tracking and integrated food databases, but I'm not a big proponent of these migraine-inducing behemoths. First, entering data can be time-consuming since you often have to search through massive databases for exact food matches. Second, many online food journals and apps place a big emphasis on counting calories or other macronutrients. All this tabulating misses the point. If you're eating mostly healthy, whole foods, such as fresh fruits, veggies, whole grains, nuts, seeds, and lean proteins, there's really no reason to get so fixated on the numbers. Plus it's just plain tedious and can often lead to unhealthy thoughts and behaviors, such as the urge to purge or a desire to repeatedly thump your head against a cement wall.

Instead, I prefer that my clients keep a simple written/typed journal or create a basic spreadsheet journal. Personally I prefer the spreadsheet option because I find it allows for easier pattern recognition. You can find an example of the food tracking spreadsheet I use with my clients in Chapter 10, as well as some recommendations for some of the more user-friendly food journaling apps.

- **Daily tracker.** If you prefer a low-tech method, you can print my "Daily Tracker" template to record your weekly wellness behaviors. Simply list your self-healthy action steps for the week and then mark the box after you complete each one, or leave it blank if you don't. See the sample below.

You can download a blank copy of this template at **jillginsberg. com/templates.**

DAILY TRACKER							
Action steps	MON	TUE	WED	THUR	FRI	SAT	SUN
1. Eat one serving of dark leafy greens per day	x	x	x	x	x		x
2. Limit simple carbs to two servings per day		x	x		x	x	
3. Exercise 30 minutes per day	x	x	x	x	x		x

- **Custom trackers.** I'm a big fan of devising my own tracking tools. For instance, take my Magical Energy Scale—a basic 1 to 10 scale, with one being "I'm practically dead" and 10 being "I'm jumping off the walls and everyone around me wishes they were dead." All you have to do is track your energy levels by ranking where you fall on the scale each day.
- **Fruit and Veggie Tracker.** This is an another example of a self-made tool. Instead of relying on memory, which can often be faulty, you can simply cross it off the page each time you consume a serving of fruits or veggies. You can find this tracker in Chapter 8.

What's most important isn't which tracking mechanism you use but that you find one that is easy for you to consistently keep up with. However, beware of becoming a tracking junkie! Track just enough to stay accountable. But don't drive yourself crazy.

Creating Your Weekly Self-Health Tracker

Monitoring and accountability go hand in hand. Having daily tracking tools keeps you focused on your day-to-day behavior, but you also need a tool that allows you to easily track your goal performance each week. That's where your weekly Self-Health Tracker comes in!

To create your Weekly Self-Health Tracker:

1. Start by entering your six-month goals and/or action steps in the appropriate section of the tracker template. Sometimes it may make more sense to track your action step instead of your goal, if your goal happens to be something that isn't easy to measure on a weekly basis. For example, if your goal is "Within six months I will have a blood pressure reading of 120 over 80" then you will be better off tracking the action step "Drink a fresh fruit smoothie every day," until you have the chance to check your blood pressure levels at your next physical.

2. When creating your Weekly Self-Health Tracker, your unit of time is one week. Determine what you should have accomplished in that first week, according to the goals you set, and enter this in the "target per week" column.

3. At the end of the week, enter your actual results in the "actual per week" column. Refer back to your various tracking tools for this data.

4. Then perform a weekly "variance analysis" by comparing the behaviors you targeted with your actual results. The variance is the difference between your target and actual results and can be positive or negative or neutral. The results of your variance analysis will tell you whether you are hitting, surpassing, or falling short of your target goals.

5. As each week progresses, continue to update your Weekly Self-Health Tracker with the one-month, three-month, and six-month goals you entered on your SMART Goals Form.

Sample Self-Health Tracker
You can download a copy of this template at **jillginsberg.com/ templates**.

Weekly Self-Health Tracker			
Goal/Action Step	Target per week	Actual per week	Variance
I will learn how to cook one new healthy meal per week for the next three months.	1	1	0
80% of the groceries I purchase each week will consist of fruits, veggies, and other whole foods.	80%	50%	-30%
I will lose 12 pounds in 12 weeks.	1	1.5	+0.5
I will add 30 minutes of movement to each weekday for three months.	150	135	-15
I will drink a fresh fruit smoothie every day	7	6	-1

What Happens When You Are On Track?

Just as businesses provide bonuses or other incentives to their employees for a job well done, you can and should reward yourself upon successfully completing a goal. You may not be able to give yourself tickets to the Luxury Box at the next Major League Baseball game or extra "paid time off," but there are lots of other ways for you to acknowledge your self-healthy achievements. A reward system not only provides you with a well-deserved pat on the back for staying on track, it also keeps you motivated to keep at it.

When my clients achieve their goals, I like to encourage them to select a bonus from my "High Five Rewards Roster." It's easy. Just reward yourself according to the level you feel is best suited to your accomplishments. I like to think of "Standard High Five" rewards as a bonus for achieving all your weekly goals, "Double High Five" rewards as a bonus for consistent achievement of your weekly goals, "Jumping High Five" rewards as a bonus for consistently surpassing your weekly goals, and "Super Fancy Fist Bump" rewards as a bonus to cash in once you've successfully completed your main goal in its entirety. But one of the perks of being a grown-up is that you get to decide what you want when you want it. So choose the reward method that works for you.

I encourage you to use your rewards as you earn them. But occasionally it's also nice to save them by putting the money you would spend on the reward into a rainy day jar or fund or underwear drawer. Then you can let it accumulate and cash it in for an extra-special reward when you feel like it.

HIGH-FIVE REWARDS ROSTER

STANDARD HIGH FIVE	• try good smelling lotions, oils, or shampoos
	• take a long, hot bubble bath
	• buy fresh flowers
	• buy movie tickets
	• buy a new make-up item
	• buy a new pedometer
	• go get a manicure
	• buy a new magazine
	• take a nature walk
DOUBLE HIGH FIVE	• go get a pedicure
	• schedule a massage or spa treatment
	• sign up for a fun new fitness class
	• try a new bottle of wine
	• buy a book
	• download an album
	• get a new pair of jeans
	• go hiking or kayaking
	• try a healthy new restaurant
	• take a yoga class
	• CREATE your own
JUMPING HIGH FIVE	• subscribe to a magazine
	• get a new pair of shoes
	• purchase new workout gear
	• get a new hairstyle
	• schedule a girls/guys night out
	• sign up for a cooking class
	• buy a new cookbook
	• CREATE your own
SUPER FANCY FIST BUMP	• pay someone to do the yard work, housecleaning, or whatever
	• sign up for a weekend retreat
	• take a day off work
	• buy a new kitchen appliance
	• CREATE your own

Other Important Considerations When Analyzing Your Self-Health Tracker

- *Convert your unit of time, when necessary.* Notice that when I entered "I will add 30 minutes of movement to each weekday for three months" into my tracker, the target amount of minutes is 150 minutes instead of 30. This is because I was calculating how many minutes I planned on exercising per week, not per day. Remember, the unit of time is one week and I am considering weekdays only for this example. There may be times when you need to convert your metric from a daily one into a weekly one. Don't be scared off by the grade-school math. You've got this!

- *It all comes down to the bottom line.* If you miss a couple of planned 30-minute workouts due to an unexpected fire drill at work, it may seem like you are way off track. But at the end of the week, what matters most is the bottom line, not what happens on any one given day. For instance, if you miss two workouts that you had scheduled earlier in the week, add a 45-minute workout to your calendar later in the week. If you can do this, you're still doing great overall and the end result is that you are only 15 minutes off of your weekly target. Not a bad end result! Or if one of your objectives is to drink less alcohol, your goal might be to "Consume no more than four alcoholic beverages per week." But perhaps you get carried away one night while karaoking with the guys from the office and you drink three "Berry White" cocktails, hoping they will make you sing more like Barry White. Sadly, the drinks don't make you sound any better but they do succeed in putting you over your allocated target by two drinks. The good news is you can get right back on track by not allowing yourself any more alcoholic drinks for the remainder of the week.

- *Consider the "Metric Matrix."* Performance metrics are most useful when analyzed as a group. Reviewing your total performance for a week shows areas of success as well as areas of weakness. Over time, this Metric Matrix approach can reveal trends and identify where you can take steps to improve your performance. For example, if you notice a pattern of not fulfilling your cooking-related goals, it may mean that you need a different healthy eating strategy. Or if you notice that you aren't meeting your fitness goals, perhaps it's time to consider a new form of exercise.

What Happens When You're Not on Track?

If you are truly challenging yourself, you aren't always going to be on track. That's perfectly fine, and there's no reason to worry if you occasionally fall short of your goals. But if you find yourself behind the eight ball, and your actuals are consistently not keeping pace with your targeted goals, here are a few points to consider.

- ***Develop a plan for improvement.*** After tracking the data for a while, you will notice which goals, if any, are weak areas for you. As long as you know what you want your metrics to be, you can come up with an improvement plan. Start by reviewing the wellness strategy that formed the basis for your action steps. This is the area you are likely having trouble implementing. Reevaluate your strategy and correlating action steps and try a different approach for achieving the same goal. For example, your goal may be "I will eat a healthy, balanced lunch every day for the next 30 days" and your strategy may be "Pack my lunch for work." But if you've noticed that after two weeks you have only packed your lunch twice and you don't have a great explanation for not packing your lunch the other eight days, you might want to instead adjust your strategy to "Purchase a healthier lunch" and make your goal "I will order a green salad every day for lunch."

- ***Adjust your target as needed.*** Sometimes it's the target, not the execution, that's out of line. You may need to modify your expectations if you're having a challenging time meeting your targeted goals. Consider extenuating factors the may be impacting your performance. Sometimes different circumstances require a different approach. If you're going through a particularly difficult or busy time, it's important to stay accountable to your self-health, but you also want to keep the importance of flexibility in mind. For instance, perhaps you set a goal of "eating three servings of vegetables every day" and your strategy is to focus on dark leafy greens. One of your action steps is to drink a green juice or smoothie every day, but suddenly you have to go out of town for a week to help care for an ailing aunt. She happens to live thirty miles from a grocery store, and the veggie pickings are slim to slimy. It won't kill you to leave your juicer at home and stick with good-old fashioned broccoli for a while.

- ***Freeze spending if needed.*** In the business world, sometimes companies have to freeze spending to get back on track. Similarly, you may need to cut off certain behaviors until you feel like you are back in control. For example, if your goal is to have only one low-calorie dessert per day and you eat the whole box of SkinnyCow ice cream treats in one sitting, you might have to eliminate dessert altogether for a week to reclaim your self-control. It's a more extreme measure, but sometimes that's exactly what's required. Especially if you're even considering licking envelopes to get your fix!

Understanding where and why you are falling short of your goals is just as valuable as knowing what behaviors are going well for you. Tracking your performance and progress will help you stay accountable to your self-healthy goals and can even help you refine your goals along the way.

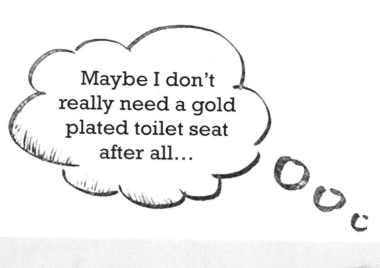
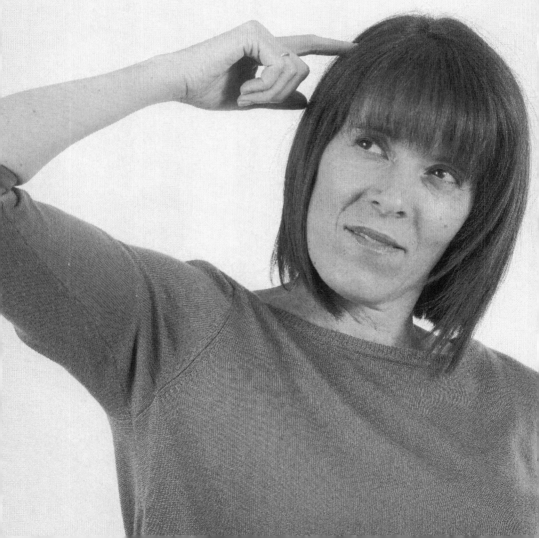

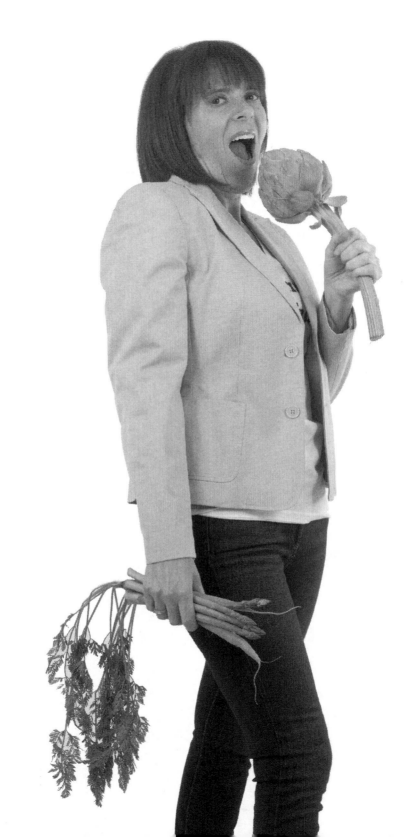

PART THREE:

LIVE LIKE A WELLIONAIRE

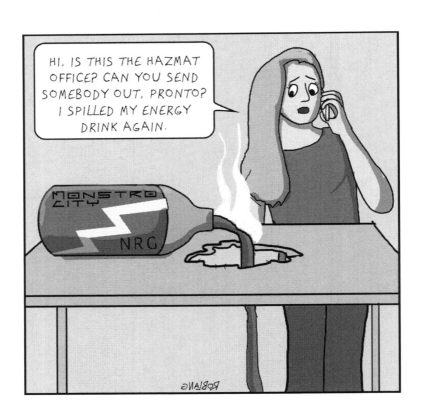

CHAPTER 9

Find Your Power-Savings Mode: Maximizing Your Energy

It's fitting that energy is defined as the capacity to do work, because without energy we wouldn't even be able to stay awake on the job, let alone be constructive.

Sadly, many of us aren't exactly killing it in the productivity department. Instead, we're experiencing a chronic energy shortage caused by longer work hours, more responsibility, and greater stress than we've ever known before. Perpetually sleep-deprived, overburdened, and undernourished, we're barely scraping by.

I've been there myself! Not that long ago, between my soul-sucking full-time job, two-hour daily commute, and a house full of adorable but needy children, I was so fried that when I saw a gym mat I wanted to lay down and take a good, long nap. Forget push-ups or bicycle crunches! If I had any spare energy left at all I might be motivated enough to create a comfy little makeshift pillow out of one of those courtesy gym towels. Cue the Muzak, and lights out. Only once I started putting my Self-Made Wellionaire principles into practice was I able to fortify my energy reserves, cast off my chronic fatigue, and reclaim my health.

Energy maximization is the most important wellness area you can focus on. Without it, you can't run your life like a boss. Hell, you can't even run at all. Energy allows you to function well at work and at home and is a necessary component for achieving other self-healthy goals and behaviors. Energy gets you to the gym and keeps you awake while you're there. It propels you to take the time to prepare a healthy meal. It keeps you focused and alert so you can maintain the mental stamina necessary to make the most of every day.

We all need energy to stay focused and alert so we can maintain the mental stamina necessary to get the most out of every day. Are you enjoying your time with your kids, or are you contemplating adjusting the clocks forward to fool them into thinking it's bedtime already? (Not that I've ever done that.) Are you competently knocking out those work projects, or are you covertly staking out your next "power nap" spot in the supply room closet? Do you manage to squeeze in an awesome sweaty workout, or is it just another day when you didn't quite get around to taking those sneakers out of the box yet?

Low energy is a common daily battle for many of us. But it doesn't have to be that way!

Just Ask Peter

You might recall Peter, one of our examples from earlier in the book. Peter said:

I want to have more energy because I'm sick of dozing off in meetings and I'm worried I'm going to get canned. I see myself waking up feeling alert and naturally being able to stay energized throughout the entire day.

Peter's related strengths included:
- Liking to sleep. A lot.
- Being home at a reasonable time.

Peter's related weaknesses included:
- Watching TV until the wee hours of the morning.
- Waking up in the middle of the night thinking about work projects.

Peter identified some improvements he could make, including:
- Going to bed earlier.
- Learning how to be more Zen.

Peter also identified the threats that could prevent him from achieving his goals:
- Regularly binging on Netflix and often falling asleep on the couch.
- Having a super-stressful job.

Peter already did most of the hard work when he formulated his vision and performed his SWOT analysis. He identified that too much television and work stress were interfering with his sleep and draining his energy.

Now go back and look at your vision and SWOT analysis. What clues can you find about what is draining your energy?

The Wellth of Energy Equation

It's easier to see the clues that are draining your energy when you understand exactly what gives you energy in the first place. Many variables impact your ability to feel vibrant and alert.

To help my clients understand the factors that most influence their energy levels, I created a trusty little formula I like to call the Wellth of Energy equation.

Wellth of Energy Equation

$$[\text{NUTRITION} + \text{EXERCISE} + \text{SLEEP}] - \text{STRESS} = \text{MAXIMUM ENERGY}$$

Simply put, to maximize your energy you want to increase the quality of your nutrition, exercise, and sleep while decreasing your exposure to stress.

It also stands to reason that the opposite equation is then true. The lower the quality of your nutrition, exercise, and sleep and the more stressed you are, the lower your energy. I like to call this one the "Land of the Living Dead" equation.

Land of the Living Dead Equation
[CRAPPY FOOD + NO EXERCISE + HARDLY ANY SLEEP]
+ PILES OF STRESS =
MINIMAL ENERGY

This, unfortunately, is the formula many of us are operating under, and it explains why so many people like Peter are walking around like soulless corpses.

Throughout this chapter we'll discuss each component of the Wellth of Energy equation in a bit more detail so you can say adios to the land of the living dead!

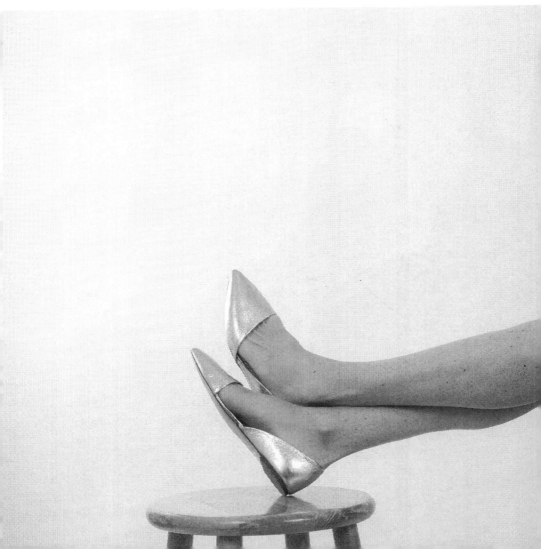

Knowing Where to Start

Most people will start to see big improvements in their energy levels with just a few small lifestyle changes at a time.

Let's turn back to Peter. He now has the missing piece to accomplishing his goal of energy maximization: nutrition + exercise + sleep – stress = energy maximization. For Peter, the two factors that are impacting his energy levels the most are sleep (or lack thereof) and stress. If he creates some action steps around sleep improvement and stress management, he should see a quick improvement in his energy levels.

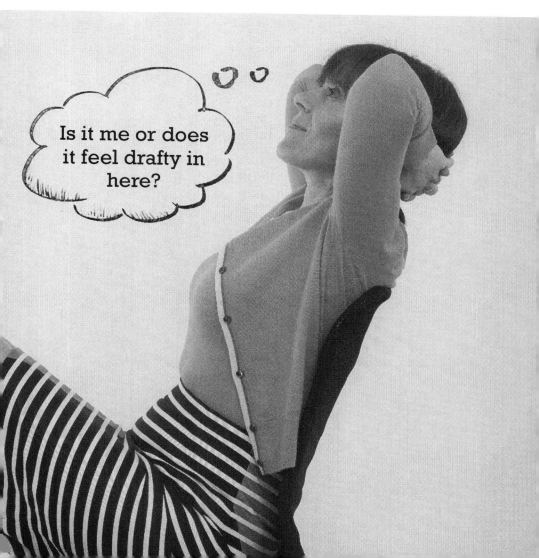

Are You Borrowing Energy?

Don't confuse natural energy with borrowed energy. If you have natural energy, you wake up feeling refreshed and stay fueled all day long without the need for any stimulants. This state is easier to achieve than you might imagine! Yet more often than not, many of us rely on "energy loans" to get us through the day. We look to things like caffeine to get us going in the morning. Then we turn to sugar or more caffeine to help stave off the infamous 3 o'clock slump.

Taking out energy loans may work in the short term, but it doesn't come without a price. Just as is the case with any loan, borrowing energy creates debt. You can only borrow so much before you completely tax your body's resources and reach your limit.

The best way to know if you're living on borrowed energy is to conduct an "Energy Audit."

JILL'S ENERGY AUDIT:
Place an "X" next to the statements below that are true for you

1. ____ I typically get less than 7 to 8 hours of sleep per night.

2. ____ I often wake up feeling tired instead of refreshed.

3. ____ Don't try to talk to me until I've had my morning cup/carafe/gallon of coffee.

4. ____ I didn't know breakfast was still a thing.

5. ____ I rarely exercise more than three times a week.

6. ____ I often eat lunch at my desk or standing up, if I bother to eat it at all.

7. ____ I tend to experience at least one "energy crash" throughout the day.

8. ____ I need a pick-me-up in the afternoon to help me stay conscious.

9. ____ I tend to doze off in meetings or whenever I make contact with a couch.

10. ____ I frequently find myself feeling irritable or impatient with my kids or coworkers.

11. ____ I rarely drink more than five 8 oz. glasses of water per day.

12. ____ I skip meals throughout the day.

13. ____ I don't have at least one hobby I participate in regularly.

14. ____ I can't remember the last time I really laughed at something.

15. ____ I have a hard time meeting deadlines.

16. ____ I don't regularly spend time with friends and family, at least not while awake.

17. ____ I often crave chocolate or something sweet, especially in the middle of the day.

18. ____ I yawn throughout the day, even around people who aren't boring.

19. ____ I sometimes use sleep aids to help me get my zzz's.

What's Your Energy Score?

If you answered yes to five or more of these questions, you could definitely stand to increase your natural energy reserves. Pronto! Keep reading to learn what you need to do to turn your body into a fatigue-fighting dynamo.

Five Strategies for Maximizing Your Energy

There are five key areas you want to focus on when trying to put some pep back in your zombie step. Even though Peter is going to be focused on the last two strategies since his biggest energy suppressors are a lack of sleep and excess stress, he'll still want to pay close attention to all the strategies, since there are a lot of interdependencies.

1. **Eat Energy-Boosting Foods**

   We all learned in school that energy comes from the food we eat. If only it were really that simple! It's true that what you eat can give you a boost. But food can also deplete your energy, depending on the choices you make.

Foods that give you a big nutritional bang for your buck include:

- *Low-glycemic/high-fiber foods.* Low-glycemic index foods release energy over time, resulting in a smaller change in the blood sugar level and a steadier, longer-lasting feeling of energy. Examples of low-glycemic/high-fiber foods include whole grains, legumes, nuts, seeds, berries, leafy green vegetables, and cruciferous veggies, such as cabbage or cauliflower.
- *Protein-packed healthy fats.* Essential fats called omega-3 fatty acids are total brain boosters and improve your mood. When you combine them with protein, it's like landing a one-two knockout punch in fatigue's face. Great sources include cold-water fish (like salmon, cod and halibut), avocados, nuts, and seeds. Chow down on avocados, raw nuts, and seeds regularly, and eat fish rich in omega-3 up to three times per week.
- *Raw foods.* Cooking food destroys nutrients and some of the enzymes that help with digestion and absorption. There's no need to swear off cooking! Just try adding more raw foods to your diet to increase your nutrient load and give your digestive system an occasional break. Raw foods include fruits, veggies, sprouted nuts, seeds, legumes, and grains.
- *Superfoods.* Including one or two superfood powerhouses in your daily diet is a sure way to amp up your energy. Examples include acai berries, chia seeds, dark leafy greens like kale or chard, and sea vegetables such as green algae and seaweed,

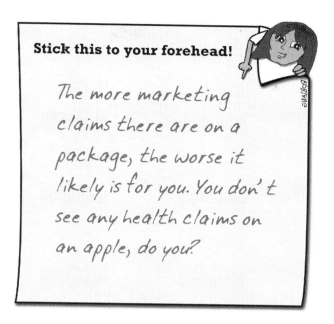

Stick this to your forehead!

The more marketing claims there are on a package, the worse it likely is for you. You don't see any health claims on an apple, do you?

among many more. Just be sure to check your teeth regularly for seeds and other miscellaneous plant life.

2. **Avoid Energy-Draining Foods**

The second strategy for maximizing your energy is to avoid draining foods. If your system has to work harder to digest food, you're using up energy, instead of gaining it!

Examples of energy-zapping foods include:

- *High-glycemic foods.* High-glycemic foods may give a quick burst of energy soon after eating them as your blood sugar rises, but it dissipates just as fast, resulting in an energy slump. Research the Glycemic Index online to see exactly which foods rank highest. Examples include the usual sugar-laden, simple carb suspects, such as soda, candy, pasta and pastries made from white flour, and sweetened fruit juices.
- *Stimulants and alcohol.* Stimulants such as caffeine, sugar, and alcohol may seem to give an energy boost, but they actually

deplete your body, drawing out minerals, water, and nutrients. Alcohol places an extra burden of detoxification on your already overworked liver. This isn't to say you need to swear off happy hour forever. Just be mindful of how that drink may be impacting your energy and sleep.

- **"Energy drinks."** Big blasts of energy never last long. Red Bull may give you wings. But, boy, when those little wings suddenly stop a flappin' and you come crashing down, the end result ain't pretty.

Food Sensitivities and Allergies

Food allergies or sensitivities can be extremely fatiguing because they cause stress and result in inflammation throughout the body. This fatigue is exacerbated by the fact that food intolerances interfere with healthy digestion and absorption of nutrients. So, ironically, even if you are eating lots of great energizing foods, you may still suffer from malnutrition and exhaustion.

Some of the more common food allergens include wheat, dairy, soy, nuts, corn, and eggs.

Food allergies usually present themselves with obvious physical symptoms almost immediately, such as hideous hives or, say, suddenly dropping dead from anaphylaxis.

But symptoms of food sensitivities are often far more vague and can occur many hours or even days after eating the suspect food. That delayed reaction can make food sensitivities much harder to diagnose. There are usually fairly obvious clues though, at least to the trained eye. If you frequently experience any unexplained symptoms such as putrid gas, bloating, skin conditions, strange rashes, warts, lethargy, headaches, brain fog, depression, or joint pain, there's a good chance you have a food sensitivity. Or you're dying. Either way, get checked out on the double!

- **Processed foods.** Filled with refined grains, fake sweeteners, and artificial ingredients, processed "foods" love masquerading behind colorful packages, wrapped in health claims that try to convince us how nutritious they are. Not only is the good stuff usually stripped out during the manufacturing process, all sorts of artificial colors, preservatives, and a potpourri of toxic chemicals are added. Talk about a double-whammy drain on your energy.

Identifying and eliminating even one food intolerance can make such a tremendous impact on your energy and health. Take it from me. I eliminated gluten six years ago. When gluten went out the window, so did my chronic fatigue, a lifelong battle with constipation, severe gas, constant bloating, brain fog, excess belly fat, and about 80% of my bitchy attitude. I've never felt or smelled better!

If you suspect you may have a food sensitivity, schedule an appointment with a health coach or physician. They can help you sort through your symptoms and, if necessary, systematically guide you through an elimination diet. An elimination diet works by removing all culprit foods from the diet and then reintroducing them one at a time. Depending on how many foods are excluded, the process typically takes about a month to complete.

Don't panic if there are several foods you need to remove during your elimination diet. There are lots of awesome alternatives for common food allergens that will make you feel like you're not missing a thing!

Food allergy testing is also available. But nothing beats the first-hand evidence you get from an elimination diet done right!

3. **Make Movement and Exercise Part of Your Daily Life**

The third strategy for maximizing your energy is to exercise. Movement is a great way to increase your energy level and fend off fatigue. Even 20 minutes a day of low-intensity exercise can transform how you feel.

I totally get that when you're already feeling five minutes away from being hospice-bound the last thing you want to do is gear up for a jog around the block. But, contrary to what most people think, exercise doesn't make you tired. It actually gives you a surge of energy... and who couldn't use a little more of that?

Exercise also makes you feel better by:

- *Lifting your mood.* Exercise releases hormones that relieve stress and promote a sense of well-being. It also lifts your mood by releasing endorphins, those much-lauded chemicals in the brain that energize your spirit and make you feel like Oprah just gave you a free car.
- *Making you feel more mentally alert.* As your heartbeat quickens, more blood surges through the brain, more oxygen is absorbed by your cells, and you feel more mentally alert and energetic. In other words, after a workout you might actually be able to help your fifth-grader with his algebra homework.
- *Helping your body work more efficiently.* Better-conditioned muscles also make daily tasks easier. When you exercise, you increase your ability to recruit and use muscle fibers so you require less effort to perform basic physical tasks, like climbing stairs, sweeping the floor, or striking those naked mirror poses you think nobody knows about.
- *Keeping you regular.* Regular exercise definitely makes you... well, more regular. One of the best ways to keep things moving on the inside is to move your body around. Ever wondered why older people get so constipated? Turns out that too much sitting around in one of those easy chairs doesn't make it so easy to go number two.

Chapter 12 is all about fitness. There are lots of specifics on how you can ease into exercise and get started, no matter how tired you may feel. Check it out for fun ideas and simple ways to incorporate more movement into your life.

4. Get Quality Sleep

The fourth strategy for maximizing your energy is to get quality sleep consistently. We've all heard how better sleep helps maintain weight, memory, energy, and sanity. But try telling that to the looming work project that's hanging over your head and infiltrating your nightmares. Or the toddler who has a brand-new big-girl bed and thinks it's hilllllarious to barge into your room. Every. 15. Minutes.

Sleep interruptions happen. Especially when you're stressed. Or procreating. Or Peter.

You can't control all the extenuating variables that might interfere with your sleep. But you can experiment with some tried and true tips:

- *Stick to a sleep schedule.* We're all really just a bunch of pre-schoolers walking around in big-kid clothes. Just like when you were a wee one, your body still responds well to routine. Going to bed and getting up at the same time every day helps reinforce your sleep-wake cycle by training your body to find its natural rhythm.
- *Create a bedtime ritual.* Perform the same relaxing activities each night before bed to cue your body that it's time to call it a day. When you're ready to get down and drowsy, dim the lights. Take a warm bath or shower. Throw on some calming tunes. Or, if all else fails, read a few pages of your old physics textbook. That ought to knock you right out.
- *Turn your room into a sleep cocoon.* Aim for cozy. Use blackout shades and get rid of digital devices that give off ambient light. Get earplugs or a noise machine to help tune out potential disturbances. Make sure your mattress and pillow feel comfy. Lastly, if they're interfering with your sleep, remind little people and pets that they have beds of their own. Or try growling ferociously. I hear it works on both two-legged and four-legged children.
- *Be mindful of what you eat and drink.* Drinking too much of anything before bed is a guaranteed middle-of-the-night trip to the bathroom. Caffeine and alcohol can disrupt your sleep, too. The stimulating effects of caffeine take hours to wear off and can keep you from falling sleep. And even though alcohol might make you feel tired at first, it commonly disrupts your sleep later.

You also want to try not to overeat or consume foods that could cause indigestion. Better still, try eating foods that put you in the mood to snooze.

5. **Minimize Stress**

The fifth and final strategy for maximizing your energy is to minimize stress. Think about how your body reacts under stress. Your muscles tighten up, your gut wrenches, your heart rate increases, your breathing becomes shallow, your pits sweat, and you may even get ulcers. Imagine how much energy your body need just to cope with all of those bodily functions! That's why it's crucial to manage stress whenever possible:

- *Minimize chemical stress.* This includes nutritional stress from the food you eat, as well as nicotine, caffeine, alcohol, and even sugar. It also includes exposure to pesticides, pollution, and other environmental toxins found in our air, water, and food supply.

Seven Sleep-Promoting Foods

These seven foods will have you snoring faster than your grandfather's old war stories:

1. **Almonds.** Almonds contain magnesium, the relaxation mineral. They're also high in protein, which means your blood sugar will stay good and balanced while you're sweet dreaming about winning the lottery and hiring that super-fancy personal chef. Try a tablespoon of almond butter or a small handful of whole almonds to help your body and brain chillax.

2. **Milk.** Milk contains tryptophan and is high in calcium, which calms the brain. Dairy not only helps you sleep, it stops you from stressing over silly stuff you can't control, like the unfortunate text you just sent to your boss in your sleepless stupor: "I hope you enjoy coming with your wife this weekend." Coming. Camping. Same difference. Warm your milk up for an extra soothing effect or add a teaspoon of honey for a deeper dose of drowsy. And relax... you'll probably still have a job in the morning.

3. **Oats.** Complex carbs like oats give you a little burst of energy followed by a crash. And since you're looking to get some serious shuteye, crashing is exactly what you're going for. Oats are also rich in vitamin B6, an anti-stress vitamin, and melatonin, the famous sleep-regulating hormone. So snag an oatmeal raisin cookie and a glass of milk, or fix yourself a bowl of steamy gruel and you'll soon be on your way to Shangri La La Land.

- **Reduce mental stress.** This includes emotional stress and often results from an imbalance in your personal or professional life. Lots of things can drain you emotionally, like work stress, a bad relationship, over-commitment, emotional vampires, annoying family members, or the ever-morbid evening news (turn it off!). Once you identify the source of the drain, you can plug it and replace it with something more positive.
- **Avoid physical stress.** This includes any form of bodily inflammation, structural problems, pain, or sickness. Exercise smart. Know your limits. Schedule a massage. Get help from health professionals. Take warm baths. Protect your immune system. Show your body some love and do everything you can to keep it safe and stress free.
- **Practice self-care.** Self-care isn't just about brushing your teeth or washing your hair. It's about nurturing what's within you. By cutting back on unnecessary activities and allowing more

4. **Whole-grain toast with honey.** Like oatmeal, wholegrain toast is rich in complex carbs that spike your blood sugar and ultimately trigger the release of the relaxation chemicals tryptophan and serotonin. The natural sugars found in honey give your insulin levels an extra boost and allow those feel-good chemicals to easily enter your gray matter.

5. **Rocky Mountain oysters.** Otherwise known as ball testicles, Rocky Mountain oysters probably won't do crap for your sleep. Just checking to see if you're still awake, seeing as you're so sleep-starved. Gotta keep you on your toes!

6. **Cherries.** Cherries are one of the only natural food sources of melatonin. Tart cherries contain higher levels of melatonin, so pucker up and embrace the sour. Throw back a shot of pure cherry juice or chow down on some fresh, frozen, or dried cherries to help direct your body to dreamland.

7. **Bananas** are loaded with potassium and magnesium, nature's happy little muscle relaxants. They also contain more of that calming tryptophan, which, ironically, can keep you from going bananas in the first place. Toss one into your blender with some milk and you'll be good to go... to bed.

time for ones that renew and inspire you, you can recharge your energy and reduce stress. Try walking in the woods, swimming in the ocean, watching clouds, or scribbling in one of those adult coloring books that seem to be all the rage these days. Oh, and feel free to grab a cheese stick or a naturally sweetened juice box while you're coloring. (Do you need help with the straw?)

Chapter 13 offers a much more extensive look at how to manage stress and provides some fun ways to practice self-care. Read that chapter if you feel like you could use some help in the not-pulling-your-hair-out department.

Creating an energized life is about balancing all the key areas of wellness, including nutrition, exercise, sleep, stress management, and self-care. When these things are all in harmony, you won't have any problem running your life like a boss.

How to Apply This Information

To begin increasing your energy:

1. Start by remembering the energy equation:
   [NUTRITION + EXERCISE + SLEEP] – STRESS = MAXIMUM ENERGY

2. Then review your vision statement and SWOT analysis for clues as to your energy drains.

3. Focus on the one or two components of the equation that are draining your energy the most. For Peter, these were sleep and stress.

4. Based on what you learned in this chapter, identify your strategy and create your Action Plan.

See some sample actions steps for improving energy below:

Sample Action Steps Peter Might Take:
- Research calming bedtime rituals.
- Order and install blackout shades.
- Turn the television off by 9 p.m. each week night.
- Read Chapter 13 of *Self-Made Wellionaire* to learn specific stress-reduction tips.

Other Sample Action Steps To Help Maximize Energy:
- Drink tea instead of my morning cup of coffee.
- Replace sugar with stevia when I bake.
- Eat fiber-rich oatmeal for breakfast each morning.
- Add chia seeds to my morning smoothie.
- Include a serving of raw veggies with my lunch.
- Drink five 8 oz. glasses of water per day.
- Do 10 minutes of aerobic exercise when I get up in the morning.
- Take a break every three hours at work and get outside for some fresh air.

You're not done yet! To create a wellth of energy, you'll want to carefully read and apply each chapter in the "Live Like A Wellionaire" section of this book. They each play an important role in the energy maximization equation!

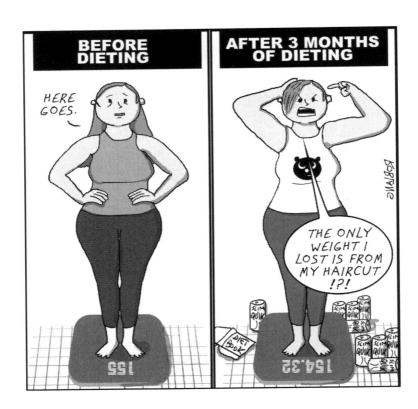

CHAPTER 10

Diversifying Your Food Portfolio: Upgrading Your Eating Lifestyle

Think of your body like a machine.

If you build it using quality raw materials, you will end up with reliable merchandise that's less likely to break down or malfunction. But if you skimp and use shoddy junk to construct your product, you'll likely wind up paying the price later when it malfunctions, breaks, or bursts into flames.

Likewise, if you fill yourself with garbage, garbage is guaranteed to come out. You will look like a hot mess. Your brain will short-circuit. Your bodily functions will be in disarray. It may not happen all at once, but eventually your input choices will catch up with you and your body will retaliate by showing signs of distress.

Whether your goal is to increase energy, lose weight, conquer cravings, lower your blood pressure, improve your cholesterol levels, become more regular, or just feel "less shitty," the food you put into your body makes all the difference.

Healthy eating is the very foundation of being a Wellionaire. Without nutritious food, no matter how many other tricks or shortcuts you have up your sleeve, your health will be subpar and deficient.

Just Ask Andy

Another one of our examples from earlier in the book featured a man named Andy. Andy said:

I want to eat better because I'm tired of feeling like a walking medicine cabinet. I see myself medication-free with my cholesterol and blood pressure under control.

Andy's related strengths include:
- He is an adventurous eater.
- He enjoys healthy foods.

Andy's related weaknesses include:
- He eats out a lot, especially work lunches, and tends to order heavier menu options.
- He's an awful cook.

Andy identified some improvements he could make, including:
- Making better choices when eating out.
- Learning how to cook.

Andy also identified the threats that could prevent him from achieving his goals:
- Frequent work travel.
- Comfort food cravings, takeout, and not stocking up on healthy groceries.

When Andy formulated his vision and performed his SWOT analysis, he identified that his reliance on restaurant food and takeout, as well as his tendency to order heavier foods, is compromising his health.

Now go back and look at your vision and SWOT analysis. How is your eating lifestyle negatively impacting your health?

A Quick Nutrition Primer

It's easier to recognize the food choices that are impacting your health when you understand some of the fundamentals of nutrition. I'm not going to bore you with endless details on recommended daily allowances or the various types of phytonutrients. Nor do I give a hoot whether or not you ever learn the proper pronunciation of zeaxanthin or quinoa. (As long as you promise to stop butchering "gyro.")

The truth is, you don't need to know any of that to start eating better. But no matter what eating lifestyle change you are trying to make, it's helpful to understand these six basic things about nutrition:

1. **Macronutrients** are important. Like really important. The word "macro" is your tip-off that these nutrients are needed in large amounts. Macronutrients include fat, protein, and carbohydrates. They provide you with energy and support essential bodily functions.
    -   Any diet or lifestyle that prohibits or limits the consumption of one or more macronutrients is unsustainable in the long run, because your body needs all macronutrients to thrive. Yup, Atkins Diet, I'm looking at you!
    -   The way to feel your best is to find the right balance, or proportion, of all three classes of macronutrients—for your body. Everyone is different. Some people feel and function better when they have more protein and fewer carbs. Others do better with less protein. The easiest way to figure out where you fall on this continuum is to experiment with different combinations of food, which we will discuss later in this chapter.

2. **Proteins** are the building blocks of life. You need protein in your diet to help your body repair cells and make new ones.
    -   Protein is found in meats, poultry, fish, grains, eggs, dairy, nuts, seeds, soy, legumes, and even in fruits and veggies.
    -   A lot of people have strong opinions (to put it mildly!) about how much protein is best. Some people swear off all animal protein in favor of plant-based foods. Other people think it's critical to have some animal protein in the diet. I say it's your body, your choice!

121

- If you include animal proteins in your diet, eat mostly lean varieties, like poultry, fish, and eggs. Be sure you're eating red meat and/or bacon only occasionally—and red meat *wrapped in bacon* even more occasionally.

3. **Carbohydrates** are the body's main source of fuel. The most common forms include fiber, starch, and sugar. Carbohydrates can be found in a variety of foods, both healthy and unhealthy, including bread, legumes, milk, corn, potatoes, cookies, pasta, and soda.
   - Carbophobia is real! Take my friend Becky. The closest contact she's had with rice in the last twenty years was when it was tossed at her during her wedding. That's because many people like Becky are confused about the benefits of carbohydrates. There are two forms—simple carbs and complex carb, and there's a big difference between the two! The types of carbs you eat matters more than the amount.
   - You want to eat mostly complex carbs, such as whole grains, veggies, beans, nuts, and seeds. Aside from being more nutrient-rich, complex carbs are also fiber-rich, which is important for intestinal health and keeping your pooper primed. Plus, since fiber gets slowly absorbed and digested by your body, it results in longer-lasting energy.
   - The carbs that you want to mostly avoid are the simple carbohydrates, which are really just sugars. Examples include white bread, pastries, sodas, and other highly processed or refined foods. Since simple carbs are rapidly digested, they cause a quick sugar spike. Then it's hello crash city! Simple carbs may make you feel good in the moment, but they'll leave you feeling down in the dumps just a short while later.
   - Fruit, although packed with nutrients, is a simple carb. To keep your blood sugar nice and stable, either opt for fiber-rich fruits like berries or apples. Or, to help slow digestion, combine your fruit with a protein, healthy fat, or complex carb. For example, try spreading a spoonful of natural peanut butter on your banana. Or dip your carrots in hummus.

4. **Fats** are essential for survival. They help us grow, develop, and absorb certain key vitamins.

- There's a myth that eating any fat makes you fat. False! You need fat to survive. You just want to make sure to eat the right kind of fat. Eating the wrong kind can indeed pack on the pork.
- Healthy fats include omega-3s, which are found in fatty fish (salmon, trout, catfish, mackerel), as well as walnuts and flaxseeds. Other healthy fats are found in olives, olive oil, avocados, coconut oil, soy, and some grain products. Eating healthy fats is actually super smart, especially if you're trying to lose weight. They keep you feeling satiated so you're less likely to go off the deep end and devour an entire package of Double Stuf Oreos.
- Unhealthy fats include trans fats and hydrogenated or partially hydrogenated oils, often found in highly processed foods such as margarine and store-bought cookies and crackers. The latest research shows that saturated fats, such as the ones found in butter, milk, or coconut oil, don't seem to be the devil they were made out to be. Enjoy them in moderation.

5. **Micronutrients** are also essential to your body and are more commonly known as vitamins and minerals. You need these in smaller amounts, hence the "micro." Examples include iron, magnesium, zinc and vitamins A, B, and C. It's pretty easy to get enough micronutrients in your diet without the need for supplements, as long as you're eating plant-based foods, such as nuts, whole grains, leafy greens, and colorful fruits and veggies.

6. **Water is the life force of everything.** You need to drink a good amount of it every day to replace the fluid you excrete. Plus, water has lots of other health benefits, like making your skin look radiant, your belly feel fuller, and your bowels function better. Although you don't have to throw back a full eight glasses a day, drink enough to keep well hydrated and quench your thirst.

The amount of water you need depends on several factors, including how active you are, the climate you live in, and your health status. If you live in a warmer climate or exercise intensely, you will need to drink more water. On the flip side, if you live in a cooler climate or eat a lot of water-rich foods, such as fruits and spinach, you will need less.

The Motivation Behind Healthy Eating

When it comes to improving nutrition, most people want to start eating healthier so they can:

- Lose weight,
- Address underlying medical issues or food allergies,
- Increase energy,
- Eliminate sugar or other unhealthy cravings,
- Learn how to make better choices and expand their eating repertoire, or
- All of the above.

When you are clear about what's motivating you to change your eating behavior, it's easier to know which strategy to implement.

Knowing Where to Start

It can be overwhelming thinking about how to best begin cleaning up your act. If you are confused about which foods are really good for you, you're not alone! Between contradictory nutrition articles rooted in pseudoscience, diet-industry propaganda, and the latest "must-try-this-so-you'll-live-to-be-an-ancient-grain" food trends, it's no wonder our bullshit detectors are going completely haywire. All the misinformation is enough to make you want to cast your chia seeds aside, smash your Mason jar meal against the wall, punch the closest Paleo person you see in the face, and drown yourself in a float pod full of refined coconut oil. Or should it be *unrefined?* Ack!

For some clarity, let's turn back to Andy. He has what are quickly becoming some serious medical issues, largely driven by his unhealthy diet. There are three main factors that are negatively impacting his nutrition:

1. Andy is dependent on outside food sources and restaurants.
2. He lacks knowledge about healthier menu and grocery options.
3. He can't cook to save his life. Literally.

If Andy forms his action steps around sourcing healthier foods and learning some basic home food preparation techniques, those should go a long way toward helping him get better. Or he could just get married! Kidding... though he probably *would* eat better.

Five Strategies for Eating Right

Here are five strategies you want to focus on when trying to upgrade your eating habits:

1. **Keep it real.** This one's pretty simple, but it's often the hardest one for people to get! Eat as many fresh, whole foods as possible. The fewer crinkly bags and cardboard boxes you have in your grocery cart, the more real your diet will be. Think about:

   - *Getting fresh.* There's a difference between an apple vs. apple pie vs. apple-flavored Air Heads. The more unprocessed it is, the better off you'll be. Opt for the freshest version.
   - *Counting on convenience.* Don't be a martyr. There's no shame in taking shortcuts whenever available. Pre-washed or precut veggies will save your butt. It's worth spending a little extra money for the sake of making "healthy" more convenient.
   - *Upgrading it.* We all begin building our foundation of wellness at a different place. If you haven't eaten a piece of fruit in so long you practically have scurvy, transitioning to whole foods is going to be harder for you. The most important thing is to begin by making small but meaningful changes to your diet. Apply the Good/Better/Best principle. This approach encourages you to make one small upgrade at a time. Aim for good at first. Then, once you have that down, try for better. Ultimately, you want to shoot for best. For instance, if you've been eating Frosted Flakes every morning for fifteen years, you might take the following approach:
     - Good: Add 1/4 cup of berries to your Frosted Flakes.
     - Better: Add 1/4 cup of berries to Corn Flakes.
     - Best: Add 1/4 cup of berries to steel-cut oats.

     Or when eating out, you could try the following approach:
     - Good: Add a green salad to your standing pizza order.
     - Better: Add a green salad to your whole-wheat pasta order.
     - Best: Add a green salad to your order of grilled chicken or fish.

- ***Eating a rainbow.*** Brightly colored fruits and veggies are packed with nutrients. Try to eat at least five servings per day, such as berries, spinach, carrots, and peppers. Use the Fruit and Veggie Tracker on the next page to check off the number of servings you have per day.

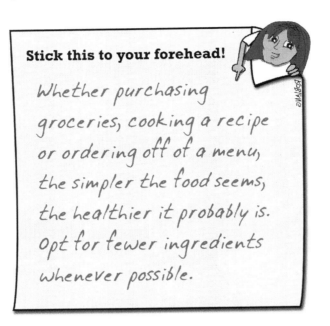

Stick this to your forehead!

Whether purchasing groceries, cooking a recipe or ordering off of a menu, the simpler the food seems, the healthier it probably is. Opt for fewer ingredients whenever possible.

Fruit and Veggie Tracker

One serving of fruits or vegetables is generally equal to 1/2 cup. Keep in mind that a proper portion of dried fruit would be less than 1/2 cup. since fruit shrinks when it dehydrates, whereas a serving of raw leafy greens would be more than a cup since it is loosely packed. It can get confusing, so to clear things up check out **www.buzzle.com/articles/ serving-size-of-fruits-and-vegetables.html.**

Each time you consume a serving, cross it off using the daily charts on the next page. Record your consumption for two weeks.

1 2 3	1 2 3	1 2 3	1 2 3
4 5 6	4 5 6	4 5 6	4 5 6
7 8 9	7 8 9	7 8 9	7 8 9
10	10	10	10

1 2 3	1 2 3	1 2 3	1 2 3
4 5 6	4 5 6	4 5 6	4 5 6
7 8 9	7 8 9	7 8 9	7 8 9
10	10	10	10

1 2 3	1 2 3	1 2 3	1 2 3
4 5 6	4 5 6	4 5 6	4 5 6
7 8 9	7 8 9	7 8 9	7 8 9
10	10	10	10

1 2 3	1 2 3
4 5 6	4 5 6
7 8 9	7 8 9
10	10

2. **Experimentation.** Businesses often like to test new ideas on a small scale before they take big risks on a wing and a prayer or commit significant resources to a project. By opening themselves up to risk in a controlled way, companies can save face and avoid larger-scale screw-ups in the future. (Remember "New Coke"?) Running simple food experiments on yourself is also a smart way to gain evidence about what does and doesn't work well for you. It helps you understand how food makes you function and feel, so you can fine-tune your choices to better suit your body's needs.

Different combinations of foods can make you feel amazing, horrible, or anywhere in between. Are you more focused or practically brain-dead when you don't include protein with your meal? Does raw garlic turn your gut into a putrid, festering cauldron of foulness? The only way to really know is to experiment with your food.

Here's how I recommend going about conducting effective food experiments:

- *Choose which type of meal/food group you are going to test.* I suggest starting with breakfast. If you can figure out which breakfast foods are ideal for your body, it will get your day off on the right foot and keep you from getting trapped on a hellish blood sugar rollercoaster ride for the rest of the day.
- *Decide what your test variables are going to be.* You can try eating low-carb, high-carb, low-fat, non-fat, meat-centric, vegetarian, or vegan. The point is to try a multitude of combinations so you can see how they impact you.
- *Identify your evaluation metrics.* Examine the effect of your food on your energy levels, your digestion, and your mood. You also want to determine the frequency in which you check in with yourself. Are you just testing how you feel immediately after eating, or do you want to consider how you feel a couple of hours later, too? I recommend doing both.
- *Record your findings.* Notice how the different combinations of macronutrients make you feel. Do you run out of steam if you don't have any healthy fat? Do you feel overly stuffed if you have too many carbs? Pay attention and a lot will be revealed.

Other Considerations When Conducting Food Experiments

There are a couple of other points to keep in mind when conducting food experiments:

- *An apples-to-apples comparison matters!* To get accurate data, you want to keep other variables constant. For instance, if you don't typically drink coffee, you shouldn't have any during the week you are conducting your breakfast experiment. You may end up writing down "energized! really! really! energized!" after eating boxed cereal and attribute this to your bowl of Cheerios when, in fact, it's really the result of introducing caffeine into your diet. Similarly, if you pull an all-nighter to binge on that latest Netflix series, you won't know if your energy is flat because you didn't sleep or if breakfast has anything to do with it. To get the cleanest results, change one variable at a time.

- **_Apply your findings!_** Learn from your findings and apply them to your future breakfast, lunch, dinner, and snack choices. Now that you know raw garlic doesn't do you right, you know to switch up your pesto recipe. If you discover that you need a mixed balance of macronutrients, then an avocado, tomato, and lettuce sandwich on whole-grain bread might be a great lunch option for you. Or if you find that your morning waffle leaves your stomach growling an hour later, try topping it with some natural almond butter and banana slices to see if that makes you feel full longer.

Try the Breakfast Experiment

Explore eating a different breakfast every day for a week. Using the template below, note what you eat and how you feel, both right after eating and again two hours later. Take a minute to sit quietly after you eat and reflect. Record how your energy level, your moods, and your physical symptoms are affected by what you eat.

You can download a copy of this template at **jillginsberg.com/ templates**.

Here's a sample breakfast experiment menu. Tailor your menu to suit your preferences—just be sure it has a good mix of options.

Day 1: Whole-grain cereal with milk
Day 2: Greek yogurt with berries and flaxseed
Day 3: Oatmeal
Day 4: A blueberry muffin
Day 5: Spinach omelet with buttered toast
Day 6: Whole-grain toast with natural peanut butter and banana slices
Day 7: Fresh fruit smoothie

Day	What I ate	How I feel right after eating	Two hours later
Day 1			
Day 2			
Day 3			
Day 4			

Day	What I ate	How I feel right after eating	Two hours later
Day 5			
Day 6			
Day 7			

Conduct a similar experiment for lunch or dinner if you feel like you need more data.

Four Ways You'll Pay for Skipping Breakfast

Skipping breakfast is a dim-witted way to start your day. Without breakfast you are more likely to be:

1. **Sleepy.** The right breakfast foods contain the important vitamins, minerals, and nutrients you need to jumpstart your day. If you don't refuel your body, it won't be long before fatigue sets in and you're flakier than Ally Sheedy's scalp in "The Breakfast Club."

2. **Grumpy.** You won't just be lacking energy. Low morning blood sugar also means low patience, which means you're far more likely to fly off the handle when your son drags his feet getting out the door in the morning. Then a couple of hours later, as you're still beating yourself up over what a horrible parent you are, your body will start sending you little craving signals to help lift your energy. The sugar rush/short-fuse cycle will start all over again, just in time to reunite with the kids. How fun!

3. **Absent-Minded.** Most of us have a hard enough time trying to remember whether or not we put on our deodorant. We don't need any help in the forgetfulness department. So if your morning is going to involve short-term memory tasks such as, oh, trying to remember whose library book is due when, which after-school activity your daughter has today, or what the hell you're supposed to say when it's your turn to present your monthly numbers to the executive team, you might want to tuck into a little breakfast.

4. **Childish.** Stop whining about how you're not hungry and how people keep telling you not to eat when you're not hungry—and start thinking for yourself. It's called "break-fast" for a reason. After not eating all night, your brain and body require food to function well. This doesn't mean you have to eat a huge meal. Drink a smoothie. Poach a freaking egg. Just suck it up and take a few bites of something reasonably nutritious.

You wouldn't send your kid off to school on an empty stomach, would you? So show yourself the same consideration and, for the love of all that is holy, eat some damn breakfast with your coffee.

3. **Follow the "80/20 Rule."** In business, the 80/20 rule states that roughly 80% of the effects come from 20% of the causes. For example, 20% of the workers produce 80% of the results while the rest of the clock-suckers are reading blogs called "How To Slack Off at Work and Get Away With It." Or 20% of customers create 80% of the revenue. The business world totally geeks out on the 80/20 rule. Knowing which customers produce the majority of their revenues is a big flippin' deal. Then management knows who to suck up to and where to focus their resources. For our purposes, we're turning the traditional 80/20 rule on its heels. But our version is just as useful! It's all about moderation and fostering sustainable eating habits. The Wellionaire's version of the 80/20 rule means committing to eating nutritious foods 80% of the time and allowing yourself to relax a little the other 20% of the time.

   • Whether you decide to make your timeframe a day (I will make 80% of my food choices healthy today) or a week (I will let myself loosen the reigns a bit during the weekend) isn't really so important. Just give yourself permission to have some wiggle room so you don't panic when you cross paths with an irresistible brownie. That brownie might find its way into your belly. But it will mostly be surrounded by yummy whole foods.
   • This rule also applies when eating out. Make lean protein, fresh veggies, healthy fats, and whole grains 80% of your meal. But order a glass of wine or a light dessert if you want.

4. **Ditch the diet mentality.** I'm a fan of four-letter words, but *diet* happens to be a four-letter word I just can't get behind. Not only do diets not work, they usually only end up making things worse! The National Institutes of Health estimates that dieters can expect to regain two-thirds of lost pounds within a year. These same dieters can expect to regain all of their weight, and possibly more, within five years. How much does that suck? Millions of people are restricting calories, fighting a daily battle with their willpower, feeling dissatisfied, and essentially hating life... only to end up being fatter than they were before.

Instead of yo-yo diets and deprivation, follow these tips:

- **Add in to crowd out.** Too often we frame making healthier food choices in a negative light by thinking about what we need to remove. That's not fun at all! Don't torture yourself by taking away all the foods you enjoy. Instead, focus on adding in healthier choices. They will naturally crowd out some of the unhealthy stuff. For instance, instead of going on a sudden sugar detox, first try adding naturally sweet foods like beets, carrots, and sweet potatoes to your diet to curb those cravings.
- **Cook more.** Cooking at home saves money and allows you to control your portions and ingredients. Even if you hate cooking, learn how to prepare a handful of no-brainer, shortcut meals using healthy, prepared foods. Anyone can cook some brown rice, heat up a can of black beans, and slice an avocado and tomato. Even Andy! There are a lot of simple, balanced, practically-do-nothing options that can become your go-to staples, no matter how inept you are in the kitchen.
- **Understand the key drivers of your "hunger."** When you're starving for affection or a deeper sense of purpose, it's easy to reach for food to try to fill the void. But food can never replace other forms of nourishment lacking in your life. If you're hungry for a more satisfying career or more fulfilling relationship, feed them. Not yourself. Paying attention to your mood when you think you're hungry can help shed light on what's really driving your appetite.
- **Right-size your portions.** In the business world, when a company's size is disproportionate to its profitability, in an effort to cut costs and become more efficient, management may decide to reduce the work force to the "right size" by getting rid of the dead weight. Similarly, if you want to get closer to your right size, portion control is a great place to start. Now more than ever before, people are experiencing a hostile takeover of their ass(et) and thighs. A lot of what's driving the obesity epidemic is the increasing size of portions. To right-size your portions, aim

to make half of each plate fruits and veggies, or serve your food on a smaller plate when eating at home. When eating out, order small plates or appetizers instead of entrees, share a meal, or ask to have half of your food boxed up.

- **_Eat regularly._** You already know that skipping meals causes your energy, mood, and hunger levels go out of whack. It's also true that waiting too long without eating will switch your body into survival mode, eventually sending you hunting with your fork and knife (the modern-day version of the bow and arrow) to quickly score some venison. Or pie. Or all the pies! Restricting calories in the short term almost always leads to binging.

- **_Keep a food journal._** Counting calories is a waste of brain cells. Instead keep a basic food journal to increase your accountability and help you get real about what you're consuming. Be as detailed as possible by including all of the ingredients you eat and the approximate portion sizes. An example of the food tracking tool I use with my clients is featured on the next page. You can add in additional rows to record the quality of your sleep, energy, digestion, mood, stress, or whatever else you feel is important to measure.

You can download a copy of this template at **jillginsberg.com/templates**.

If you prefer to use a food journaling app, check out *MyFitnessPal* or *Lose It!* Both have user-friendly interfaces, which make them the perfect choice for food journaling newbies.

WEEKLY FOOD JOURNAL

	MONDAY	TUESDAY	WEDNESDAY	THURSDAY	FRIDAY	SATURDAY	SUNDAY
Date	1/31						
Breakfast	Green smoothie with spinach, 1/2 banana, frozen berries, almond milk, and protein powder						
Lunch	2 slices of gluten-free avocado toast with sprouts; 1 hard-boiled egg						
Dinner	Roasted lemon artichoke chicken, 1 cup of steamed broccoli and 1/2 cup of wild rice						
Snacks	1/4 cup of dark chocolate almonds, two baby oranges, cucumber slices, and 1/4 cup of hummus						
Drinks	Earl Grey Tea; Water						
Water	1 2 3 4 5 6 7 8	1 2 3 4 5 6 7 8	1 2 3 4 5 6 7 8	1 2 3 4 5 6 7 8	1 2 3 4 5 6 7 8	1 2 3 4 5 6 7 8	1 2 3 4 5 6 7 8

5. **Be Mindful.** You already know that paying attention to what you put into your body matters. But it's equally important to pay attention to *how* you put food into your body. So often, we eat mindlessly. We don't even remember what or when we ate because we're so busy doing everything else at the same time. Tune into the eating experience:

- *Eliminate distractions.* Turn off "Parks & Recreation." Put the computer and your phone away. It's okay. All of your "Friends" will still be there when you're done. Well, except for the three who "unfriend" you for not immediately liking their latest status update. But anyhow... sit down, settle in, and savor your food without distractions.
- *Chew your food well.* We're in such a rush to get everything done, eating is often just another thing to cross off our to-do list. We forget about the importance of actually chewing! Chewing helps your body to digest food and absorb nutrients. There's nothing like trying to chew each bite thirty times to make you realize that you've been swallowing your food whole your entire life. See, there is a reason we have teeth!
- *Slow down.* We've all heard that it takes about 20 minutes for the brain to register that the stomach is full. By slowing down your pace of eating and taking the time to taste, smell, and enjoy your food, you'll feel full and satisfied on less food. Take one bite at a time, put your fork down, and remember to breathe. Or try one of my favorite slowing-down tricks... chopsticks!

How to Apply This Information

To begin improving what and how you eat:

1. Start by reviewing your vision statement and SWOT analysis for clues about how your eating lifestyle is negatively impacting your health.

2. Focus on the one or two areas that are most impacting your nutrition. For Andy, the factors most impacting his nutrition are his dependence on outside food sources and restaurants, his lack of knowledge about healthier menu and grocery options, and his lack of cooking experience.

3. Based on what you learned in this chapter, identify your strategy for healthier eating and create your action plan.

Sample Action Steps Andy Might Take:

- Drink a fresh fruit smoothie every day.
- Pack a healthy lunch for work on Monday, Wednesday, and Friday.
- Sign up to receive daily recipes from a blog that specializes in using five ingredients or less.
- Bring a fresh piece of fruit to work to eat as a snack every day.

Other Sample Action Steps to Upgrade Your Eating Lifestyle:

- Conduct the Breakfast Experiment (see page 129).
- Buy pre-washed and sliced veggies for lunches and snacks.
- Chew each bite 30 times during dinner.
- Use the Fruit and Veggie Tracker to record servings (see page 127).
- Start using a daily food journal.
- Purchase smaller plates and begin using them for meals.
- Sign up for a healthy cooking class.
- Include a vegetable with dinner every night.
- Order a lighter dish from the appetizer section of the menu instead of a full entree.

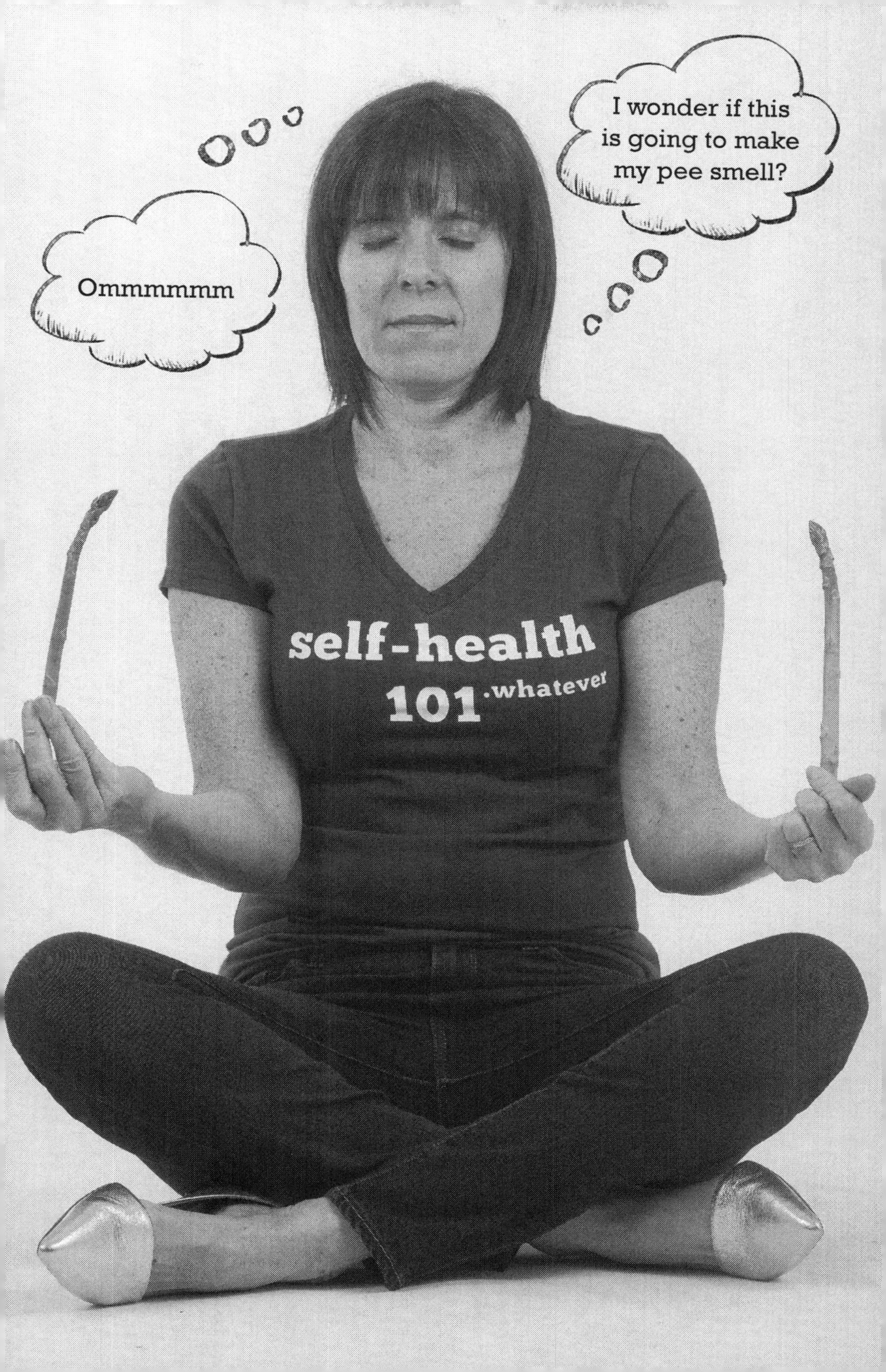
I wonder if this is going to make my pee smell?
Ommmmmm
self-health
101·whatever

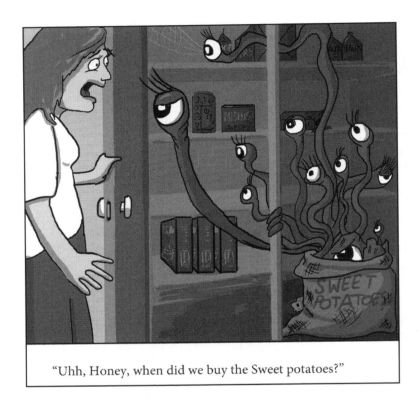

"Uhh, Honey, when did we buy the Sweet potatoes?"

CHAPTER 11

Hedging Your Bets in the Kitchen: Meal Preparation Principles

An effective manager doesn't head into the office on Monday and ask, "Now what?"

She already knows her next steps because she has a plan. With deadlines looming and projects that need completing, a plan is necessary to make sure that money, resources, and customers don't fall through the cracks.

Similarly, if you want to effectively manage your nutrition you don't head home Monday night and say "What's for dinner?" The infamous six o'clock scramble (it's no accident the initials spell out SOS) is a real-life nightmare that repeatedly plays itself out in homes across America and around the world. You're tired. The kids are hungry. Everyone's running on empty and nobody has a clue what's going to end up on the kitchen table 30 minutes later. Pretty much the only thing you know for sure is that somebody's going to have a total mental breakdown. It might be one of the kids. It might be you. Unless he's lucky enough to already have gone deaf, it might even be the family dog. If you have a picky eater or someone with food sensitivities, the situation is only exacerbated. Now, instead of trying to come up with one last-minute meal idea, you're scrambling to come up with two or three.

All the stress around meal time is enough to make you want to stick your kids on the corner of a busy intersection with FREE signs dangling from their necks, march yourself down to the nearest airport, and hitch a one-way ride to Anywhere But Here.

Or you could plan ahead.

Just Ask Maria

Another one of our examples from earlier in the book featured a woman named Maria. Maria said:

I want to be more regular because I'm sick of pooping once a week and feeling like a bloated cow. I see myself feeling lighter and having one good bowel movement a day.

Maria's related strengths include:
- She enjoys lots of fruits and veggies.
- She has a Costco-sized package of toilet paper just waiting at the ready.

Maria's related weaknesses include:
- She has a hard time giving up foods she loves.
- Her middle name might as well be Dairy.

Maria identified some improvements she could make, including:
- Eliminating foods that are messing with her digestion.
- Finding substitutes for the foods she will miss the most.

Maria also identified the threats that could prevent her from achieving her goals:
- The rest of her family members don't have food sensitivities and her kids don't like change.
- Lasagna. Enchiladas. Omelets. Pretty much everything she cooks for her family has cheese in it. She's worried that she won't have the willpower to cook something separate for herself, and she doesn't have time to prepare multiple meals to try to please everyone.

When Maria formulated her vision and performed her SWOT analysis, she identified that some suspect foods in her diet may be contributing to her constipation. To try to meet her goal of eliminating problem foods, Maria has to adjust her diet. If she doesn't take the time to think ahead and create a meal plan that works for everyone in her family, she will end up eating the same constipation-inducing food she has in the past because it's easy and familiar. Or she'll go bonkers. Or both!

Now go back and look at your vision and SWOT analysis. How do you think meal planning might help you to achieve your wellness goals?

Stick this to your forehead!

browse cookbooks for inspiration, then, once you know what you want to cook, use the Internet as a resource to find exactly what you want. It's a lot easier to locate a great "broiled miso salmon" recipe than it is to scour the web for "great salmon recipes."

The Benefits of Meal Planning

Meal planning isn't just a sanity saver. It also helps you:
- **Be more efficient.** If you know what you're going to fix for dinner, and you have everything you need at your fingertips, getting food on the table is a cinch. It also means fewer trips to the store since you can plan your grocery list for the entire week in advance.
- **Eat healthier.** When everyone's melting down because they're starving, it's all too easy to order takeout or speed dial the pizza delivery guy. If you plan your meals and already have the ingredients you need at home, you're much more likely to prepare a quick, healthy dinner instead.

- **Save money.** A few extra things seem to magically make their way into most people's shopping carts every time they go to the store. And those things aren't free! If you shop less frequently and only for those items that you actually need, you will spend a lot less money on groceries each week. Not to mention you won't be dining out as much or relying on takeout to save the day.

- **Save time.** No more pacing the kitchen each evening for 20 minutes frantically trying to figure out what's for dinner. Everything you need to make dinner, from the recipe to the ingredients, will be right at your fingertips. Plus, as fun as it is to watch people fight with the self-checkout machines, you'll also save time with fewer grocery trips to the store.

- **Plan around preferences.** Planning ahead makes it easier to conceive a meal that the whole family can enjoy. The alternative is being a last-minute, short-order cook (also known as a short-tempered cook).

Knowing Where to Start

Meal planning isn't just for Type A folks—though, boy, does it ever make us happy! It's a necessary tool for managing your food, honoring your healthy eating intentions, and creating harmony in the house. Just think—there will be no more nagging from your kids about serving leftovers two nights in a row, you won't forget that you are having little Matthew over for dinner and try to serve him Kung Pao Chicken when he's deathly allergic to peanuts, and you'll finally get to dust off that crockpot you got for your (first) wedding.

With my simple system, once you get the hang of it, you will be able to complete a weekly meal plan in just a matter of minutes—one that includes a variety of delicious, healthy foods that even you-know-who won't whine about.

Let's turn back to Maria. She needs to change the way she eats if she wants to make Dr. Oz proud and take one good dump a day. To do that, she is going to need to start thinking ahead about her meals and snacks so that she can avoid trigger foods. If she creates some action steps around meal planning and meal preparation, she should be able to stick to her safe foods.

Four Tongue-In-Cheek Ways to Get
Your Kids to Compliment Your Cooking

Parents often have to endure hearing way too many cooking complaints and not enough compliments. Like...

"The tortillas are too soggy!"

"That oatmeal looks like a big bowl of boogers!"

"The brisket's too fatty!"

"The chicken's too dry!"

"You didn't put enough cheese in my enchiladas!"

"There's a bone in my fish ... ewwwwwwww!"

Sure, you could employ all sorts of strategies to encourage your children to be less persnickety. Like offering more variety at meals. Or more ketchup. Or more ranch dip. Or more bribes.

But these tired techniques don't really give kids an appreciation for all the wonderfully healthy food you've already been trying to feed them. Sometimes you just have to reach for something a little more clever, like these four tips:

1. *The school cafeteria.* If you're a lunch packer like me, you're going to want to bury those adorable little bento boxes in the back of your cupboard where dust bunnies go to die. This week your lucky kiddo is dining on school barfaroni, rubbery chicken nuggets, and mystery meat, with a side of rodent droppings. Bon appétit! They'll be good and hungry by the time you serve dinner.

2. *Meal Ready to Eat (MRE).* Give your little one an MRE for dinner and let them pretend they're in the military for the night. Since MREs can be heated without a fire or stove, little Johnny can have a warm meal in the comfort of your home without you having to cook or worry about anyone burning the house down. Then he can wash his gray stew and spreadable "cheese" down with a tasty powdered beverage mix. Mmm mmm delicious. If it's good enough for the military...

3. ***Dumpster diving.*** It's time for your kids to find out what it feels like to be a freegan. Join a Meetup group if you must (they have them!) and jump on the dumpster-diving trend. Supermarkets across the nation toss perfectly good meats, cheeses, eggs, and produce into the trash every day. Your kids might get lucky and find a veritable feast. Bonus tip: Turn it into a learning experience and make sure to highlight the abhorrent food waste problem we have in our country.

4. ***Back of the freezer.*** You know all that unlabeled shit you put in a Tupperware and stick in the back of your ice box only to be freezer burned and forgotten about? Defrost that goodness! Create a mystery smorgasbord and let your kids go to town. They'll be determined to eat it all, too, after that guilt-riddled lesson on wastefulness. I hear the Arm & Hammer Baking Soda Fridge-n-Freezer Odor Absorber makes for a nice condiment.

Even Pavlov's dogs would stop salivating after a week spent eating this crap. Give it a shot and, I promise, your kids will quickly realize just how good they really have it. Hope you have some extra Land O'Lakes lying around because they're about to butter you up.

Meal Planning Strategies

A meal planning strategy gives you a place to start. It's a jumping off point for creating your weekly menu. Feel free to experiment with any or all of these strategies when building your meal plan:

1. **Taking inventory.** Open up your pantry, freezer, and refrigerator and notice which items need to be used up. Perhaps you have a lot of potatoes that are starting to sprout and need to be eaten, a half-empty box of pasta, or a can of artichokes that you've had since you first moved in. Maybe you have some meat in the freezer that needs to be used up. Allow these ingredients to inspire your next meal! Except for the moldy salami from last year's New Year's Eve party. You can compost that.

2. **Recipe review time.** Dig out your recipes and locate those lost cookbooks because you're going to need them! Whether looking online, in a recipe folder, or through your collection of books, this strategy is all about surveying the possibilities. Look for recipes that are healthy, simple, quick, and family-friendly (if you have a family)... the fewer ingredients, the better. Compile a list of the recipes that sound good to you.

3. **Weekly staples.** This is a clever way to build variety into your meal plan with a recurring weekly theme. Try eating the same type of food on consistent days of the week. While this method allows for creativity, it also helps narrow down the possibilities so you can easily decide on a main meal idea. You can categorize your weekly staples by cuisine, primary ingredient, type of dish, cooking method, or a combination. Here are some examples:

   - Meatless Monday
   - Taco Tuesday
   - Crockpot Wednesday (not to be confused with "Crackpot Wednesdays" when you invite your eccentric artist neighbor over so you can hear his latest conspiracy theories)
   - Grillin' Thursday
   - Fish on Friday
   - Stir-fry Saturday
   - Soup and Salad Sunday

4. **What's on sale?** This strategy involves shopping the healthy savings at your local grocery store and building a meal plan based on the weekly specials. Is chicken on sale? Grab a bunch and plan a meal or two around it. Toss the rest in the freezer for another week.

5. **International mix-n-match.** Like international cuisine? Use the following chart to come up with yummy combinations. For example, if you feel like having Thai for dinner, pick out a protein, a sauce, some veggies, and a starch. Then find a recipe or purchase a healthy premade shortcut. Try making, for example, tofu with snow peas and carrots in peanut sauce served over jasmine rice.

INTERNATIONAL MIX-N-MATCH CHART

Cuisine	Protein	Method	Dishes, Sauces, and Rubs	Vegetable	Starch (optional)
Asian	Chicken	Grilled	Ginger Orange Sesame Glaze	Bok Choy	Soba Noodles
	Beef	Sautéed	Garlic oyster sauce	Broccoli Rabe	Brown Rice
	Pork	Stir Fried	Teriyaki Sauce	Carrot	Rice Noodles
	Tofu	Kabob	Black Bean Sauce	Green Bean	
	Fish	Broiled	Sweet and Sour Sauce	Mushroom	
Italian	Chicken	Grilled	Fresh Basil Pesto	Tomato	Pizza Dough
	Beef	Broiled	Fennel and Crushed Red Pepper	Sweet Onion	Polenta
	Pork	Sautéed	Basic Italian Seasoning	Eggplant	Risotto
	Beans	Roasted	Lemon Juice and Olive Oil	Bell Pepper	Pasta
	Fish	Poached	Ragout (Pasta Sauce)	Zucchini	Beans
Indian	Chicken	Braised	Curry Rubbed	Cauliflower	Basmati Rice
	Lentils	Grilled	Coconut Curry Sauce	Tomato	Potatoes
	Pork	Sautéed	Cilantro Mango Chutney	Peppers	Brown Rice
	Lamb	Kabob	Vindaloo (Spicy Curry)	Spinach	Sweet Potato
	Fish	Broiled	Tikka Masala (Tomato Sauce)	Okra	Lentils
Thai	Chicken	Grilled	Green Coconut Curry	Onion	Jasmine Rice
	Beef	Sautéed	Red Curry Rubbed	Tomato	Thin Rice Noodles
	Pork	Braised	Lime and Lemongrass Soup	Peppers	Black Rice
	Tofu	Roasted	Peanut Sauce	Snow peas	Wide Noodles
	Fish	Broiled	Yellow Curry Sauce	Carrot	
Latin American	Chicken	Roasted	Chipotle and Tomato Sauce	Corn	Refried Beans
	Beef	Broiled	Cilantro Salsa Verde	Tomato	Black Beans
	Pork	Grilled	Fajitas	Sweet Onion	Pinto Beans
	Fish	Braised	Enchiladas	Peppers	Rice
	Beans	Stewed	Adobo Sauce	Avocado	Tortillas
	Beef	Roasted	Carolina or St. Louis BBQ Rub	Tomato	Potato

INTERNATIONAL MIX-N-MATCH CHART					
Cuisine	Protein	Method	Dishes, Sauces, and Rubs	Vegetable	Starch (optional)
American Regional	Chicken	Grilled	Cajun Gumbo	Corn	Tortilla
	Pork	Broiled	Southwest Chile, Black Bean, and Corn	Sweet Onion	Bread
	Fish	Poached	Rosemary Roast with Apple-Cranberry Stuffing	Peppers	Beans
	Beans	Braised	Pineapple-Soy-Ginger Marinade	Braising Greens	Rice
French	Fish	Sautéed	Roasted	Carrot	Bread
	Chicken	Braised	Poached with Fine Herbs and Leeks	Shallots	Potato
	Beef	Poached	Bourguignon	Green Beans	Lentils
	Pork	Roasted	Stuffed with Mushroom and Goat Cheese	Leeks	Celery Root
	Beans	Broiled	Tomato, White Bean, and Garlic	Peas	Vegetable Gratin

Jill's Top Meal Planning Tips

Before you begin, there are some classic organizational business tips to keep in mind that will help you make the most of your meal plan:

- *Have a set weekly meal planning time.* Pick a consistent day of the week and time to create your meal plan. This will help meal planning become a habit. Plan before you shop.
- *Be smart about where you start.* It's beneficial to plan out all your meals. But, if you're not up for tackling every meal at the outset, I recommend starting with dinner. By the time it rolls around, people are usually fed up and beat from their busy day. So it's the time you're most likely to take shortcuts and make excuses if you don't already have a plan in place.
- *Share resources and eliminate waste.* Try to choose recipes that share ingredients in common. You won't have to buy as much variety and you'll cut back on waste by using up all of the ingredients that you do purchase. If you buy Thai basil for a curry dish, use the rest later in the week when making lettuce wraps.
- *Play to your strengths.* Try to incorporate as many tried and true recipes as possible into your weekly meal plans. Cooking dishes that you are already familiar with will save time because you already

know what to do. If you're looking to expand your repertoire, add in one new recipe each week to keep things interesting. Just cook the new recipe on a night when you have a little extra time.

- **Keep a file.** When you see a recipe you like, print it or tear it out and place it in the front of a folder with your other favorite recipes. Or, if you prefer electronic files, pin the recipe to your "Meal Planning" board on Pinterest. When it comes time to make your next weekly meal plan, your collection of recipes will all be in one place.
- **Plan seasonally.** Base meals on things that are local and/or seasonal. Usually foods that are in season are at their nutritional peak and lowest price—and they usually lack the preservatives needed to transport foods across long distances.
- **Look for economies of scale.** Quickly transform tonight's yummy dinner into something just as great tomorrow by cooking once, eating twice. Make a meal one night and use the leftovers to create a new meal the next night. For example, cook tofu stir fry one night and serve it with rice. The next night use the leftovers to make baked tofu enchiladas. You'll keep things interesting, cut back on cooking time, and achieve economies of scale by making your primary ingredients work twice as hard for you.
- **Make it customizable.** Design your meals so that they are flexible enough to suit the entire family's needs. If there's a picky eater in the house, try to make meals that allow each person to customize the components, instead of mixing everything together. Burrito bars and make your own pizza nights provide enough flexibility to accommodate everyone.
- **Recycle and reuse.** Don't reinvent the wheel each week/month/year. Once you have several months' worth of meal plans in your arsenal, recycle them throughout the year. Try mixing and matching meals to create a fresh new weekly or monthly meal plan. At the end of the month you can also file that entire meal plan away until the next year. Then, you can bring it out a year later and know that you're incorporating lots of seasonal foods into your menu.

How to Create Your Own Meal Plan

These are the simple steps you will want to follow each week:

STEP 1: Write down your family's favorite meals.
Think about the recipes you and/or your family have come to love and

make a "Family Favorite Meals" list so you can reference them when making your monthly meal plans. Let these crowd pleasers be a part of your regular rotation. Add new favorites to this list each week.

STEP 2: Note important commitments on the meal planning calendar.

Get out your calendar or planner and scan the upcoming week for scheduled activities, events, and commitments, such as kids' activities, social plans, or late work nights. In the "Note" area, indicate important reminders, such as when you will be dining out, having company, or requiring a quick meal.

STEP 3: Identify the meal planning strategy or strategies you want to use.

The meal planning strategies are a jumping off point for creating your weekly menu. Feel free to experiment with any or all of the strategies. They will help you to get a jump start on filling in your plan.

STEP 4: Assign a main course and one or two side dishes for each day of the week.

Based on your schedule for the week, assign a main course to each evening you plan to cook. Then add one or two side dishes (if applicable) to accompany each main course. Remember to incorporate some of the meal planning tips, such as using shared ingredients, cooking once, eating twice, and making seasonal recipes.

STEP 5: Find recipes.

Use your recipe file, the Internet, or cookbooks to find a simple recipe to accompany every assigned main course and side dish. Avoid over-complicated, high-maintenance recipes that have tons of ingredients. Stick to recipes with five to ten ingredients, max. And sometimes a recipe isn't necessary, like if you're simply grilling chicken breast or cooking something from memory.

STEP 6: Make a shopping list.

Review your recipes and add any ingredients you don't already have on hand to your grocery list. Then head to the store and get it done! Remember, the goal is to go food shopping once per week, so you want your list to be all-inclusive.

You can download a blank copy of the following template at **jillginsberg.com/templates.**

Jill's Weekly Meal Planner (sample dinners included)		Grocery List
Monday Note:	**Friday** Note:	❏
Breakfast: Toast with almond butter and honey	Breakfast: Blueberry power smoothie	❏
Lunch: Chia seed pudding with berries and shredded coconut	Lunch: Loaded sweet potato	❏
Dinner: Tofu fried rice with zucchini, peas and carrots	Dinner: Broiled pesto salmon	❏
Side: N/A	Side: Quinoa pilaf	❏
Side: N/A	Side: Roasted vegetables	❏
Tuesday Note:	**Saturday** Note:	❏
Breakfast: Oatmeal with raisins and almonds	Breakfast: Chicken sausage, spinach and tomato omelet	❏
Lunch: Leftover fried rice	Lunch: Pasta and tomato salad with leftover pesto	❏
Dinner: Spiced garbanzo bean and cauliflower tacos	Dinner: White bean, chard and chicken chili	❏
Side: Purple cabbage slaw	Side: Cornbread muffins	❏
Side: Pickled radishes, jalapeños and avocado slices	Side: N/A	❏
Wednesday Note:	**Sunday** Note: Soccer practice	❏
Breakfast: Green smoothie	Breakfast: Gluten-free waffles with berries	❏
Lunch: Avocado, tomato, onion, and sprout sandwich	Lunch: Meeting Jen for lunch (leftover chili for the kids)	❏
Dinner: Mushroom and spinach frittata	Dinner: Roasted butternut squash and apple soup	❏
Side: Baked sweet potato fries	Side: Tomato and spinach salad	❏
Side: N/A	Side: N/A	❏
Thursday Note:	**Additional Reminders:**	❏
Breakfast: Egg-white omelet with smoked salmon and tomatoes	Make extra muffins for the potluck.	❏
Lunch: Hummus with olives, veggies, and stuffed grape leaves		❏
Dinner: Baked eggplant Parmesan		❏
Side: Kale salad and lemon vinaigrette		❏
Side: N/A		❏

Don't be afraid to switch assigned meal days around to suit eleventh-hour schedule changes or cravings. If you have all of the ingredients on hand already, you'll have the wiggle room you need to orchestrate last-minute switches.

Healthy Shopping Tips

Navigating the grocery store can be a humongous headache if you don't know what you're looking for. Keep these shopping tips in mind to fill your cart with healthy choices.

- Most of your food should come from the produce section. This is where you can find all those brightly colored nutrient-rich fruits and veggies. Aim to see a rainbow of color in your basket, including red, green, blue, purple, yellow, orange and white. The rest should come from the perimeter of the store, where other fresh foods like dairy, meat, and fish are usually located.

- Avoid the "junk sale" happening in the center aisles. Remember that when buying packaged foods, the fewer ingredients the better. If you can't pronounce or recognize an ingredient then do you really want to swallow it or serve it to your kids?

- Know when it pays to buy organic. The PLU number of Organic produce should begin with a "9." See the insert on page 155 to understand when it makes sense to pony up for organic, and when it doesn't.

- Go for lower fat meat options such as ground chicken, turkey breast or 90% lean ground beef.

- Canned fish like salmon, sardines and anchovies are an awesome source of cheap protein. Add them to pastas, salads, and dips.

- Eggs are a perfect balance of protein, carbs and fat, and they are one of the only foods that naturally contain Vitamin D. Look for organic, free range and vegetarian fed.

- Check labels to make sure you aren't getting those nasty hydroge-nated oils.

- For low-temperature cooking, try sesame oil and olive oil. For high-temperature cooking, try grapeseed oil or coconut oil. Grapeseed oil doesn't have any flavor whereas coconut oil does.

- The bulk food section is perfect for people on a tight budget or if you're cooking for one. You can get smaller amounts of low-cost grains, seeds and beans because they don't have all the fancy packaging.

- To avoid getting 12-year-old wheat germ, shop the bulk section of a well-trafficked store to ensure that the items are fresh.

- When shopping for snacks, reach for raw trail mixes or walnuts which are packed with heart-healthy omega-3 fatty acids. Low-fat popcorn is also a good whole-grain, high fiber choice. Make dark chocolate with 70% or more cacao your sweet craving savior.

- Canned kidney, black or pinto beans are rich in protein and fiber and make a hearty addition to salads, soups and dips.

- Watch out for hidden ingredients in canned veggies and fruits. Sugar and sodium are often added.

- Opt for whole-grain breads, rolls or tortillas. They'll stick with you longer and keep you feeling satisfied.

- Stock up on a few convenient nutritious foods for days when all hell breaks loose. Pre-portioned and pre-marinated tofu, fish filets or chicken breasts, shelled edamame and healthier frozen meals, such as Amy's brand products, are great last-minute back-up options.

- Incorporate frozen fruits and veggies when the seasons don't allow you to include some of your fresh favorites. Frozen fruit is good for blending year-round smoothies and frozen veggies make easy additions to grain bowls or stir-fry dishes.

Stick this to your forehead!

After eating beans people tend to become a member of the "frequent flatulence club." To reduce the likelihood of fouling up the air, drain all liquid from the can and rinse the beans with fresh water before using them. Cooking beans with kombu (a type of sea vegetable) can also improve their digestibility and reduce gassiness.

What the Yuck! 12 Times It Pays to Buy Organic Produce

Fruits and veggies do the booty good. It's no surprise. They're filled with important vitamins and nutrients that, when balanced with other healthy foods, keep you feeling and looking your best. But they're often chock full of nasty pesticides, too.

Pesticides mess your shit up. Why do you think the insects don't want to get anywhere near 'em? Pesticides are linked to cancer, birth defects, nervous system damage, and hormone imbalances. Studies even show that pregnant women with high levels of certain pesticides in their system gave birth to children who, years later, scored lower on IQ tests.

What. The. Yuck. A chemical smorgasbord and dumbing down our kids doesn't exactly sound wise to me. Neither does scrubbing the skins of fruits and vegetables obsessively until my fingers bleed. So what's a well-intentioned girl to do? You can certainly reduce the number of pesticides in your life—and your body—by purchasing organic fruits and veggies. But buying all organic all the time may not be something you can afford.

The trick is knowing when you need to buy organic and when you can afford to get away with the conventional varieties of fruits and veggies.

Luckily for us, the Environmental Working Group (EWG) publishes two annual lists, based on their research, which takes all the guess-work out of it. Be sure to look for an updated list each year. The EWG points out helpful tidbits, like the fact that 99 percent of apple samples tested positive for at least one pesticide residue. First it was Eve. Then Snow White. Now it seems the apple continues to earn its spot as the most vile fruity villain around. But apples aren't the only concern. Even a single grape can carry as many as 15 different pesticides.

Here's the EWG's 2015 list of the fruits and veggies with the most pesticides—known as the "Dirty Dozen":

1.   Apples
2.   Peaches
3.   Nectarines
4.   Strawberries
5.   Grapes
6.   Celery
7.   Spinach
8.   Sweet bell peppers
9.   Cucumbers
10.   Cherry tomatoes
11.   Snap peas (imported)
12.   Potatoes

The fruits and veggies with the least pesticides—known as the "Clean Fifteen"—are:

1.   Avocados
2.   Sweet corn
3.   Pineapples
4.   Cabbage

5. Sweet peas (frozen)
6. Onions
7. Asparagus
8. Mangos
9. Papayas
10. Kiwi
11. Eggplant
12. Grapefruit
13. Cantaloupe
14. Cauliflower
15. Sweet potatoes

Buying organic whenever possible might be the holy grail. But if that's just not doable, EWG's guide can help you navigate the produce aisle like a boss. You can buy conventional versions of the Clean Fifteen and spend your hard-earned moolah upgrading conventional Dirty Dozen items to organic instead. Unless, of course, you want a family full of pesticide-laden pudding brains.

You can read the EWG's full report at **www.ewg.org** and even download a convenient app to help you remember what's what.

Stick this to your forehead!

Make cooking something to look forward to and you will want to do it more often. Turn on some tunes. Pour a glass of wine. Lighten up and have fun!

Quick Preparation Tips

Here are some business-inspired time-saving tips to manage your food preparation and work more efficiently:

- *A little extra effort goes a long way.* When cooking dinner, make a little extra for breakfast or lunch the next day. Leftover brown rice can be used as a breakfast porridge, for burrito fillings, or in a healthy fried rice. Boil some extra eggs during breakfast and—boom—egg salad it is for lunch the next day!
- *Take advantage of ready-made components.* Incorporate high-quality, ready-made ingredients. A lot of grocers have a prepared foods section with tapenades, marinated vegetables, and spreads. You can use these to season proteins, spruce up a sandwich, make bruschetta, or add quick flavor to soups. A rotisserie chicken can be tossed in with a kale Caesar salad or used to make a pot pie.
- *Use shortcuts when they make sense.* Get thin cut proteins like chicken breasts, fish, and steaks to cut back on prep and cooking time. Warm up to frozen veggies; today's processing methods preserve big flavor at the peak of freshness.
- *Batch your work.* Try chopping your vegetables for the week in advance. If you chop veggies for more than one meal you'll dramatically cut down the time spent on meal prep. Small containers of diced onion, sliced carrots, and so forth will make it easy to have items ready to be tossed into a soup or sauce. Or buy pre-washed, pre-chopped veggies. It's more expensive. But time is money too!

Quick Cooking Tips

Here are some classic everyday business tips to help you stay on your toes in the kitchen and put your best foot forward when cooking:

- *Stay sharp.* A dull knife is a dangerous knife because it is difficult to control when cutting. A sharpener or a honing steel will maintain a knife edge and make cutting easier and safer.
- *Go big.* Get the biggest cutting board that you can easily store and clean. A large work area makes cleanup easier and gives you a lot more freedom to chop and mince without worrying about food going everywhere.

- **Know what you're getting into.** Don't just read the recipe as you go along. Read the entire recipe before you begin so you can avoid unpleasant surprises, like figuring out that you just tossed an entire cup of cornmeal into your pizza dough when it was only meant to be used to help you roll the dough out. Oops!
- **Don't boil the ocean.** When boiling food like pasta and vegetables, there are three quick rules to follow to make the process easier: salt your water, more water is usually better than less, and always use a lid. The salt will help the water come to a boil faster and season your food. Using enough water lets the pot come back to a boil faster after you have added things to it. And a covered pot will come to a boil much more quickly than an uncovered one.
- **Sometimes it's good to go for the shock value.** When cooking your vegetables, bring your pot of salted water to a boil, add your vegetables and cook. While the veggies are cooking prepare a bowl of ice water big enough to hold them comfortably. Then remove the veggies from the boiling water just before they are cooked through and put them in the ice water to "shock" them and stop the cooking process. This will give you crisp, colorful, and delicious veggies every time.
- **Start with the steps that take the longest.** Get your water boiling, preheat the oven, and start first with the foods that take more time to cook. You can then move on to preparing other items. As the water is boiling for the pasta, cook your veggies. When the oven is preheating, rub your meat with spices or throw a quick marinade on your fish.

And the most important tip of all—don't be afraid to make mistakes! Kitchen blunders are often the best way to learn and will only end up making you a better cook. Pinterest porn is fun to look at, but it's enough to make even seasoned cooks suffer from extreme feelings of inadequacy. Use it for inspiration, not as a yard stick.

How to Apply This Information

To begin implementing healthy meal planning and preparation into your life:

1. Start by reviewing your vision statement and SWOT analysis to see if planning your meals and preparing ahead could improve your health. Hint: The answer is always yes!

2. Create your weekly meal plan, starting with dinner. If you desire, you can also plan your breakfasts, lunches, and snacks.

3. Based on what you learned in this chapter, identify some additional actions steps you can take to make meal planning and food preparation easier for yourself.

Sample Action Steps Maria Might Take:
- Research dairy-free substitutes online to make altered versions of family favorites.
- Stock up on pre-chopped veggies.
- Schedule time each week for meal planning.
- Buy a binder to collect recipes.

Other Sample Action Steps to Help with Meal Planning and Preparation:
- Get a magnetic grocery list to hang on the fridge.
- Go through old cookbooks and highlight recipes that are appealing.
- Buy a new cookbook that focuses on dairy-free recipes.
- Make a list of family favorites.
- Create a list of new meal ideas to get a jump start on planning.
- Make a list of easy side dishes.
- Check out the weekly grocery store circular to see what is on sale.

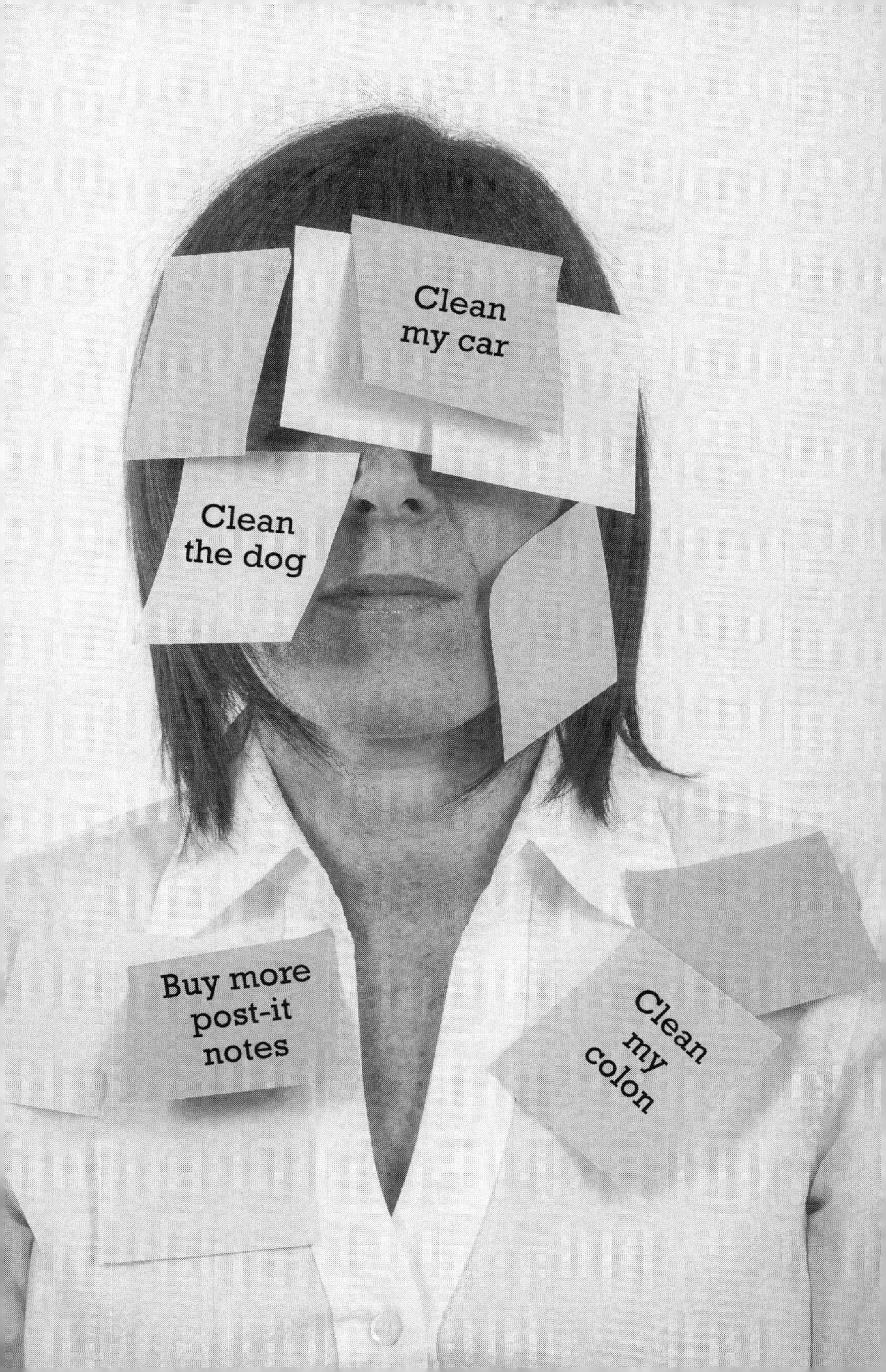
Clean
my car
Clean
the dog
Buy more
post-it
notes
Clean
my
colon

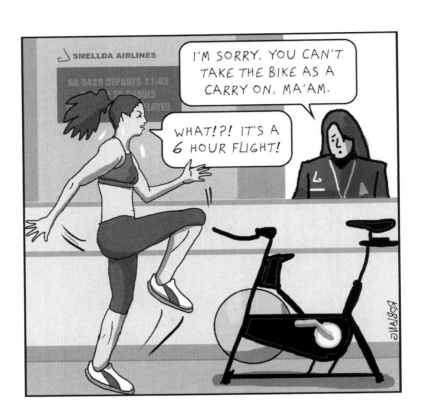

Identify Your Core Competencies: Integrating Fitness Into Your Life

In business, there is constant pressure to move faster and smarter. To gain a competitive advantage, you have to be agile.

With a growing emphasis on technological advances and a constantly evolving environment, the ability to quickly respond to changing market conditions is more essential than ever before. It's all about flexibility! When change happens or an obstacle presents itself, an agile enterprise doesn't panic and give up. Instead, it swiftly adapts to the circumstances and adjusts strategies, without losing momentum.

These adaptable qualities aren't just necessary for business success. They're important to you and me, too. Because life is a marathon every day! It's a race just to keep up with daily obligations, let alone unexpected hiccups. One of the best ways to keep your head and body in the game, no matter what kind of pandemonium unfolds around you, is to exercise.

Fitness combats stress, improves sleep, promotes endurance, and sharpens your body and mind, allowing you to be responsive to whatever life throws your way. It makes you physically more nimble and increases your mental agility, both of which are critical for Wellionaires!

Just Ask Carol

Earlier in the book we were introduced to Carol. She said:

I want to start exercising more because I'm tired of stuffing my flabby body into my clothes and feeling uncomfortable all day. I see myself fitting comfortably into my clothes and feeling secure wearing the styles I like.

Carol's related strengths include:
- She likes to be active and enjoys taking the kids hiking and swimming.
- She likes to test out new fitness classes.

Carol's related weaknesses include:
- She has a tight budget and her schedule makes it hard to get to the gym.
- She snacks all day long.

Carol identified some improvements she could make, including:
- Learning quick, effective exercises that she can do anytime, anywhere.
- Blocking out time in her schedule to exercise so that nothing interferes.
- Finding some healthier snack options.

Carol also identified the threats that could make it difficult for her to achieve her goals:
- She's a single mom who works 10 hours a day and then has to cook dinner and help her kids with homework.
- She's a nighttime snacker.

When Carol formulated her vision and performed her SWOT analysis, she identified that her limited budget and busy schedule are interfering with her desire to get fit.

Now go back and look at your vision and SWOT analysis. What factors or circumstances are hindering your ability to reach your fitness goals?

Knowing Where to Start

People tend to fall into one of three fitness camps. Either:

- **They don't exercise at all.** It's been so long, these folks think Zumba is a new-fangled pharmaceutical drug for erectile dysfunction. Typically, people in this category don't exercise because they believe they are too far gone or they have convinced themselves that they hate working out.
- **They sort of exercise.** But they are unmotivated and inconsistent, often citing time as an excuse. People in this category tend to work out in fits and bursts, especially around the New Year, bathing suit season, high school reunions, and whenever an ex announces on Facebook that they are getting married.
- **They regularly exercise.** Fitness is a consistent part of their daily routine. People in this category will find a way to get their work out in no matter what. They are so committed, if they had a broken wrist they would still knock over, with their one good arm, anyone who tries to steal their spin bike before proceeding to ride one-handed. All the more challenging!

Let's turn back to Carol. She clearly falls into the second camp. Carol enjoys working out but doesn't do it consistently. If she creates some action steps around identifying efficient workout strategies and improving her time management, she should be able to begin making fitness a consistent part of her self-healthy routine, despite her frenetic schedule.

Top Five Strategies for Getting Fit

Here are my top five strategies for incorporating fitness into your busy life, no matter which camp you fall into:

1. **Identify your "fitness personality."** When considering which job is best for you, it's helpful to know more about your personality so you can set yourself up for success. For instance, do you work better when you are the Head Honcho or do you prefer being in a structured setting with someone giving you direction? Do you like collaborating with others, or do you prefer to work alone?

Similarly, getting to know your personality better helps you understand which type of fitness is ideal for you. Identifying your "fitness personality" enables you to understand which activities most suit your preferences and keeps you from jumping on the hottest trend just because everyone else is doing it.

For instance, say your bestie purchases a 100-class punch card at the local yoga studio and swears that downward dog and tree pose are the answer to everything. So you decide to give it a try and join her, only to end up stuck in child's pose for most of the class—apropos considering you silently wept like a baby the whole time.

Or say your brother talks about SoulCycle like he's a bona fide cult member, so you decide to give the spin gym a whirl. But no more than three minutes into the workout, you begin to wonder if your soul is all that's going to be left of you because you feel like you are *actually dying.* If you weren't so breathless you would crawl over to your brother and hug him goodbye for all of eternity.

This happens to a lot of people. They try a new form of exercise only to end up frustrated, bored, insecure, or totally discouraged, sometimes even deciding that they just aren't made to work out at all!

Stick this to your forehead!

Identifying your fitness personality lets you find activities that truly suit you, so you won't end up with a closet full of Ab Rollers, ThighMasters, pogo sticks, and other assorted "latest fad" gear you used only once.

Jill's Fitness Personality Quiz

Work with your personality, rather than against it! Start by answering the following questions to zero in on the type of exercise that suits your personality and keeps you motivated. Select the answer that fits you best:

1. You enjoy exercising:
   A. Solo.
   B. With a team or group.
   C. With a teacher or guide.
   D. With whoever happens to be around.
   E. With your remote control.

2. When thinking about exercise, you:
   A. Can't wait to get going!
   B. Look forward to a little friendly competition.
   C. Want to do it but need a little shove.
   D. Like it as long as it's not too structured or formal.
   E. Dread the idea.

3. You exercise because:
   A. You have to. Without it you wouldn't feel like yourself.
   B. You see it as another way to have fun with your friends.
   C. You want to stay fit, improve your health, and/or get more swipes on Tinder.
   D. You feel like it!
   E. Your wife/girlfriend/latest obsession voluntold you to.

4. When you exercise, you prefer:
   A. Consistency. You tend to exercise at the same time and perform the same activity several days per week.
   B. Feeling connected with other people. This inspires and motivates you.
   C. Someone telling you what to do.
   D. Pretty much anything. You will happily change your workout up depending on the weather, season, or time.
   E. The easiest option possible.

5. Your idea of a great workout is:
   A. Getting your heart rate up and dripping in so much sweat you can practically see the calories spilling onto the floor.
   B. Having a fun, social time with friends while also getting in a decent workout.
   C. Tracking toward a specific goal and achieving it, such as calories burned or pounds lifted.
   D. Chasing the sunshine and going for a hike, run, or bicycle ride.
   E. Lifting and lowering beer/chocolate cake/fill-in-the-blank to your face.

Mostly As: Self-Motivator

You have no problem finding time to exercise and you function best in a structured, organized environment. Sticking to your routine is easy for you, but performing the same type of activity may leave you in an exercise rut. To challenge yourself and avoid hitting a plateau, try adding in a new activity every now and then. Or change up your workouts by adding interval training, where you alternate bursts of high-intensity exercise with short recovery periods.

Mostly Bs: Team Player

For you, exercise is a social activity that allows you to stay connected with friends. You feed off of other people's energy and enjoy motivating one another. Group classes or team activities are a natural fit for you. Sign up for an exercise class, join a running club, or register for a sports league, like softball or dodgeball.

Mostly Cs: Lead Me There

You want to exercise but you don't exactly get excited about it. If left to your own devices you will typically let competing priorities interfere and back-burner your workout. That's why you prefer when someone else is holding you accountable. You are motivated by having a set appointment with a personal trainer or a pre-scheduled time for an instructor-led fitness class.

Mostly Ds: Go With the Flow

You love freedom and spontaneity. Adventure and trying new activities motivates you. On any given day, depending on the season, you might be mountain biking, hiking in the woods, running on the beach, or skiing the slopes. Fitness isn't something you separate out from other parts of your life. It's simply a part of how you exist. You could use a little consistency, though, and would benefit from having at least one planned day of exercise.

Mostly Es: Give Me a Reason
You need a bigger sense of purpose to motivate you to exercise, other than being fit. Try planning your fitness around deadlines or larger goals. Sign up for a race three months from now that supports a meaningful cause. Then you'll have a reason to go pound the pavement. Or book an active trip, such as a cycling tour through Napa, to encourage you to start training on the bike.

The best exercise you can do is the one you WILL actually do. A huge range of physical activities exists. All you need to do is find one that suits your personality... and stick with it!

2. **Think outside the box.** If you use the excuse that you hate exercise as a reason not to bother, or the idea of working out makes you want to play dead, I have good news for you. You don't have to exercise! (This is especially relevant for those who get mostly 5s in the Fitness Personality Quiz.)

   - *Stop thinking of it as exercise!* Instead, think of it as movement and do some sort of physical activity every day. You don't need to jump on a piece of cardio equipment to get your heart rate going! A lot of people associate fitness with a sweaty 30-minute run or a 45-minute weight-lifting session at the gym, but anything that gets your heart rate going counts as fitness. Aerobic activity can include mowing the lawn, cleaning the house, or something more traditional like jogging. The ultimate key to staying fit and healthy is to find movement that you enjoy, and then do it consistently.
   - *Bring the fun!* Incorporate movement that's more recreational and makes you forget you're working out—like dancing, geocaching with the kids, or playing a game of flag football. Other fun ideas that will make you forget you're trying to be fit include:

biking, belly dancing, boxing, roller skating, ice skating, golfing, paddle boarding, rock climbing, snowboarding, surfing, and beating the pants off of your partner in a Wii sports game.

3. **Make time work for you.** Lack of time is probably the most common excuse for not exercising. Having too many balls in the air or not having enough time for fitness is not a good excuse, no matter how many hours you're logging at the office!

   - *Chunk your time.* There's a common misconception that you need to exercise for at least 30 consecutive minutes to get any health benefit. But the truth is, as long as it adds up to 30 minutes or more of moderate activity a day, that's what counts. If you don't have a solid block of 30 minutes, try breaking your activity up into 10-minute chunks at different times during the day. Do 10 minutes in the morning, 10 more minutes in the afternoon, and 10 minutes in the evening. Everybody has 10 free minutes!

   - *Remove the commute factor.* Going to the gym is great for some people. But getting there and back eats up valuable time that could be used for other activities, and this often becomes an excuse not to exercise at all. Find a few quick workouts to have on hand the next time you have a busy day. There are great "5-minute" routines you can find on YouTube. Or pop in an exercise DVD. Other great "at home" workout ideas include stairs, stationary exercise equipment, or jumping rope.

   - *Kill two birds.* If exercise is something you don't always enjoy, pair it with something you do enjoy. Combine exercise and socializing by going on a power walk with a friend, or sign up to take a class together. Or listen to an audio book while on the treadmill.

   - *Use your time wisely.* You spend all day sitting, don't spend all of your lunch time sitting too. Turn sit time into fit time. Combine your cardiovascular exercise with a sedentary activity. Hop on that piece of home equipment while watching TV or returning phone calls. At the office, go for a 20-minute walk with coworkers on your lunch break or sneak in a few squat sets at your desk (if anyone looks at you funny just tell them you dropped a paper clip). Or if you're home with the kids, walk to the playground instead of driving.

4. **Aim for quality over quantity.** The amount of time doesn't determine how effective a workout is—effort does. The trick is to be as efficient as possible.

   - *Intensity matters.* You don't need to work out for long if you use your time wisely. Maximize the intensity of your workout and get your heart rate up to make sure you get the most bang for the buck. It doesn't matter whether you are exercising for 30 minutes or 10 minutes, show up and work hard! Fitness movements like CrossFit are all about high-intensity workouts. While it's not for everyone, and I've seen a lot of people injure themselves by pushing it too far, a 10-minute CrossFit workout can bring you to your knees. Just be safe!

   - *Work out in quick bursts.* Interval training allows you to burn more calories in less time and improve your aerobic capacity. Just a couple of 30-minute sessions per week can supercharge your endurance and fitness. Or try a Tabata workout—each one is only 4 minutes, but it's liable to feel a lot longer! The workout is structured by pushing yourself as hard as you can for 20 seconds followed by 10 seconds of rest, for a total of eight rounds. You can incorporate just about any exercise you want, such as squats, pushups, burpees, or deadlifts.

   - *Get an efficient full-body workout.* Choose exercises that work all the major muscle groups. Circuit training provides both a strength and cardiovascular workout. You put several exercises that work different parts of the body together to create your "circuit." Then you perform a designated number of reps for each exercise before moving on to the next exercise in the circuit. When you complete all the exercises in the circuit, rest for 1 to 2 minutes before going through it again, typically for a total of three sets. The goal is to keep moving throughout the entire circuit with little to no rest so you maximize your time and intensity.

5. **Build in accountability.** The more accountability you can build into your routine from the beginning, the more likely you will be to stick with a fitness program.

   - *Put some money on the line.* It's amazing how forking over some cash will help you get off your butt. Trainers are the ulti-

Stick this to your forehead!

For a basic interval workout, start with a 10-minute warm-up. Then run, bike or row for 30 seconds as fast as you can. Recover for 2 minutes. Repeat each 30 seconds on/2 minutes off segment five times. End with an 8-minute cool-down period.

mate accountability tool. You have a set appointment that costs real money. Plus they also help measure your progress and keep you on track to meet your goals. Better yet, sign up for a group training program. You won't get as much focused attention or a totally customized routine, but it's a great alternative to pricey personal training sessions. Pre-paid group fitness classes are also a solid, budget-friendly option.

- *Foster teamwork.* It's easy to smack the snooze button silly when it's just you, but if you know a friend is waiting at the track for you at 6 a.m. on a Monday, you're much more likely to show up and run those laps. You can also join a team sport. Or find a workout buddy who shares your passion for cycling and sched-ule weekend rides together. You may not enjoy riding in the rain, but if he's in, so are you!

- *Set your sights on a goal.* Set your sights on a goal or sign up for a competition to keep your motivation high. Now's the time to finally sign up for that charity 5K you've been politely side-step-ping or say "yes" that to that idiotic mud run your co-worker has been nagging you to try.

- *Network.* Use an app like Fitocracy or MapMyRun, a workout tracker that ties into a social network, and you've essentially gotten yourself a virtual workout buddy. You can find workouts, log your performance, follow friends, and even compete with the community. Or try Pact, where users commit to carrying out a fitness (or other healthy) action by betting on themselves. The latter should be avoided by gambling addicts!

You can also tap into your own network. When you see annoying messages clogging up your feed, like "Heading out on an 11-mile run in the morning. Sneakers ready. Pumped!!!!!" it's not done solely to irritate you. Some people hold themselves accountable by shouting their intentions out to friends.

Other Tips for Incorporating Exercise Into Your Life

If you are just starting to exercise:

- *Start small.* Think of yourself as a startup. You need some time to ramp up and develop your stamina before you can go big. For example, if you want to start running but you're so sedentary your legs have practically atrophied, instead of starting out with the goal of running on the treadmill for 30 minutes, start by running for 1 minute then walking for 9 minutes. Do this in 10 minute increments for a total of 30 minutes. Keep increasing the number of minutes ran as compared to walked until you can comfortably run for 10 minutes straight. Then keep increasing from there!
- *Walk the walk.* Walking is as low impact as you can get, and pretty much everyone can do it! Get a pedometer or free pedometer app and record your steps. Simply notice where you are, at first, without making any changes. Then try adding on 100 steps more a day and work your way up. Eventually, you should shoot for 7,000 steps or more. The ultimate goal is 10,000 steps—equivalent to exercising strenuously for 30 minutes or walking 5 miles per day!
- *Don't be intimidated.* There's always going to be someone who knows more than you and has been doing it longer than you. But keep in mind that we all start as exercise newbies. Nobody cares that you're huffing and puffing your way up the trail or grunting in agony on the elliptical. They're all too busy looking at their phones anyhow! If you feel like you don't know enough to try something— like the TRX, for instance—ask a more experienced friend to show

you the ropes, pull an instructor aside, or sign up for a session with a trainer at your gym. Many offer free consultations to give you a chance to test them out.

- **Manage expectations.** Transformation doesn't happen overnight and not without a lot of effort. It took a while for you to get out of shape, and it's going to take a while for you to get in shape. As much as you want to see instantaneous results overnight, it doesn't work that way. To avoid discouragement, modify expectations and focus on taking it one step at a time. As long as you are consistent, you will reach your fitness goals!

If you are a seasoned exerciser, remember these "don'ts:"

- **Don't overdo it.** Don't push yourself too hard. If you overexert yourself and don't allow your body time to properly recover, it creates physical stress and drains your energy, which we talked about in Chapter 9. It's also a good way to end up burning out altogether.
- **But don't "phone it in" either.** When you stick with the same exercise routine for too long it's easy to find yourself in a rut. You may be spending 60 minutes at the gym, but if you're just going through the motions, reading *People* magazine and checking your email every 5 minutes, how hard can you really be working? Don't kid yourself into thinking that just because you are showing up, it counts. It takes a whole ass to work out. Half-assed doesn't count.
- **Don't reach the point of diminishing returns.** There's only so much cardio you can do before you're just wasting your time and energy. More work doesn't always lead to better results. You will see results at first, but eventually you will hit your plateau point and increasing the time spent exercising or adding more intensity won't help. You will only end up injured, frustrated, and fatigued. Remember the concept of "quality over quantity" and work out smarter, not harder.
- **Don't become totally predictable.** Add variety to your exercise routine. Whether it's a cardio dance class that changes choreography every week or running in a different location each weekend, if you have the tendency to get bored by routine, shake it up to keep it interesting. This will keep you and your body guessing.

Three Easy Exercises Even a Total Lazy Ass(et) Can Do

You don't have to do hundreds of military squats, train for a half marathon, or sweat smelly buckets to reap the big benefits of exercise. But if you want to stay healthy and feel your best, you do need to make exercise a regular part of your daily routine, no matter how drained you feel. It's never too late to get started, and it doesn't have to be hard. Even a total lazy head can incorporate these three invigorating, easy exercises into their daily routine. No specialized equipment, jogging trails, or pricey gym memberships required.

Stairs. Unless you live in a ranch-style house, an igloo, or a tent, I'm guessing stairs are readily available in your home or building. So start using them! The next time you run up to change that load of laundry or run down to let the dog out, take some extra trips up and down the stairs while you're already on the move. Start with ten climbs up and down. Take a break. Then tack on additional sets of ten as you need more challenge. Try skipping every other step to work different muscles. When at the office or shopping, ditch the germ-infested elevator or escalator in favor of the stairs. You work on the eighteenth floor? Ride up sixteen flights and walk up from there the first day, then keep adding on one additional flight of stairs every couple of days. Eventually you might be walking the entire way. No more awkward hum-drum elevator conversations with Tom from Accounting. *Approximate calories burned in 1 hour of Stair Climbing at a moderate pace: 500.*

Walking. Expecting a call from your chatty (promiscuous) half-sister? Throw on some sneakers and take that conversation on the road where inquiring little minds can't hear you. Vying for that perfect parking spot at Target? Stop circling the lot like a stalker and, instead, park a little farther away and walk a few extra feet. Now you can direct all of that pent-up competitive energy toward wiping the floor with your family during Friday Bingo night. Don't let the weather or your location be an excuse for not getting out there. It might be harder, but you'll burn even more calories walking in sand or snow, so look on the bright side. Grab the dog, his leash, and your flip flops, and head for the nearest beach. Or, if it's snowy, hoof it to the local sledding hill with the kids. The faster you walk the warmer you'll stay. Plus, you'll be there to witness who *really* started the snow ball fight. ***Approximate calories burned in 1 hour of walking at a moderate pace: 285.***

Household chores. If you're already vacuuming, dusting and mopping then you're also burning calories. Don't just save the tidying regimen for when your finicky mother-in-law visits. Make the household chores a regular part of your weekly routine. Your home will look better and so will you. Stagger one task on top of the other while working at a decent pace and you'll get a genuine cardiovascular workout. Amp up the fun by blasting some of your favorite '90s tunes and dancing while you clean. You'll burn even more calories. And c'mon, like you haven't fantasized about fluffing pillows while belting out Britney's "Hit Me Baby One More Time." So the next time your kid accidentally coats the windows in sticky fingerprints, thank her for helping you out, grab that bottle of Windex and put a little elbow grease into it. ***Approximate calories burned in 1 hour: vacuuming, 190; mopping, 190; dusting, 170; window cleaning, 180.***

Climbing, walking, cleaning—it all adds up to you being healthier. Playing with your kids is another great way to sneak some easy exercises into your day. So the next time junior asks you to get in on his hopscotch game, get off your lazy bum and say yes for a change. He'll be thrilled to have you participate.

See, everyone's happy when you're more active. Talk about a win-win.

Excuse/Strategy Matrix

It isn't easy to fit exercise in when you are overworked and always pressed for time. How do you squeeze more into your life when you are already drowning in responsibility? While it's true that being fit makes you more agile, it's equally true that you need to be agile to make room for fitness.

Otherwise it's all too easy to come up with an excuse not to. Why do you think millions of people make New Year's resolutions on January 1 only to end up being riddled with guilt come February? They get swallowed up by small obstacles and lose sight of their big goal, instead of responding—like an agile business would—by making adjustments or adopting a new strategy.

Use my handy matrix to find strategies to overcome the five most common excuses for skipping fitness.

Excuse/Strategy Matrix: Quit Your Whining!

1. I don't have time!	You'll have plenty of time when you're dead, which will happen sooner than you think if you don't start exercising: • Chunk your time by building in small blocks of more frequent exercise. Try 10 minutes at a time. • Plan ahead so you can manage your time more effectively and schedule windows for fitness. • Try getting up 20 to 30 minutes earlier. • Walk whenever you can. Take a brisk stroll outside during a break at work. Leave the car at home if your destination is close. • Use the stairs instead of escalators or elevators whenever possible.
2. I'm always with my kids!	Kids love being active so it's all the more reason to get moving: • If kids are a distraction, join a gym that offers childcare. Arrange a swap with a friend. Or maximize nap time—theirs, not yours. • Grab one of the other parents and walk the field at your kid's soccer game. • Work out with them! Try hiking, walking to the duck pond, biking, or kicking the soccer ball around.
3. I don't have money!	You can get a great workout without spending a dime if you are really committed to finding a way: • Get outside. Walk. Hike. Run or chase your kids around. These are all free! • Find a gnarly set of stairs to climb, either inside or outside. • Do a bodyweight workout. You can use your body's own resistance to do pushups, squats, crunches, arm dips, and lunges. • Try running. All you need is a decent pair of shoes. Plus, I hear barefoot running is a thing. • Watch (and exercise to) free online workout videos or borrow a fitness DVD from the library. • Make a small investment in two of the most versatile (and cheapest!) pieces of fitness equipment around: the resistance band and ball.

4. I'm self-conscious!	Start working out and you won't feel that way for very long: • Work out at home. Buy a piece of inexpensive gym equipment if you have the space for it, or use what you have on hand. • Hire a personal trainer to show you the proper technique and make you feel supported. • Hit the gym during off-peak hours. Or avoid gyms altogether until you are more comfortable and work out at home. • Sign up for an introductory class where you will be surrounded by others who are just getting started.
5. I'm tired!	Fantastic! Exercising is one of the best ways to give your energy a little boost so you better get started: • Commit to just doing 10 minutes at a time. Once you get going, you may surprise yourself and hang in there for longer. • Go to bed earlier to build up your sleep reserves. • Prepare your workout gear the night before so you don't have one more thing to do in the morning.

Easy Exercises An Even Lazier Ass(et) Can Do

Great news! You don't even need to get up to do these exercises. So there's really no excuse for not trying them out.

Easy Couch Exercises

No need to stop watching that "Real Wives of Hell" marathon. You can do these from the comfort of your big couch dent. Instead of fast forwarding through those commercials, perform some basic exercises until the break is over. You have about three minutes so make the most of it.

• **Start with arm extensions.** Hold a two- to five-pound free weight in each hand. Hell, hold two cans of beans, it doesn't matter, as long as it weighs something. Sit on the edge of the couch so that your arms hang straight down by your knees. Sit up nice and tall, then lift your arms straight up so they're directly out in front of you. Extend them straight out on either side of your body, forming a T with your torso, then bring your straight arms back down to your side. Now reverse the sequence by lifting your arms out like a T first, bringing them in front of you, and then back down to the starting position. Repeat 10 times.

- **Next do some tricep dips.** Sit on the very edge of the couch, balancing your weight on the heels of your feet and keeping your fingertips pointed forward. Then lift your entire body off the seat, lower it for two counts until your booty hits the floor, then rise back up to full arm extension. Don't sit down until you've done 10 to 20 in a row.
- **Finish with leg lifts.** Slowly raise one leg at a time as far as you can. Then slowly lower it back down again. Repeat 10 times, then switch to the other side. Keep adding more leg lifts every few days with the ultimate goal being 50 per side.

If you're feeling super motivated, mix these strength training exercises up with jogging in place and you've got yourself the makings of a legit workout. Look at you go!

Easy Car Exercises

You might not enjoy being in the car as much as you love being parked on your couch, but between all that commuting, the kid's gazillion extracurricular activities, and the endless list of errands to run, you probably spend plenty of time sitting in traffic. While you're waiting for the gridlock to clear up, try this simple routine. It sure beats watching the guy next to you pick his nose like he's digging for a three-carat diamond.

- **Tighten that butt.** Engage and release your glutes 20 times in a row, holding your cheeks tighter for 10 seconds and then releasing for 5 seconds. Rest for 45 seconds and then repeat. They don't call 'em butt pinchers for nothing!
- **Work that core.** It's easy, just act like you're yawning (which should be very familiar to you), raise your arms straight up above your head, and place your hands against the roof of your car. Push up with your arms and squeeze with your abs at the same time. Hold for 10 seconds and release. Repeat as many times as you can. To challenge your core even more, try lifting one or both of your feet off the ground (just don't forget to put your car in park first).
- **Get your groove on.** This one needs no explanation. Just dance like nobody's watching (even though they are definitely watching) for one full song. You'll feel amazing and you might even lift the spirits of those around you. Are they smiling at you or laughing at you? What's the difference, really? You just made their day.

Easy Bed Exercises

These easy exercises are perfect for truly lazy people since there's no need to even get out of bed. Hell, you barely need to toss off your crumb-littered sheets:

- **Pretend you're riding a bike.** Lie on your back, bend your legs up toward your chest and pedal your feet in a circular motion. You should feel your abdominal muscles begin to tighten. When it starts to hurt, stop. Rest. Then do it again two more times.
- **Scissor kicks.** Stay in your horizontal happy place, put your hands underneath your low back, extend your legs out, and lift your shoulders off the bed slightly. With your legs extended and flexed, open and close them repeatedly like a scissor without letting them hit the mattress. Continue for 30 seconds.
- **Small crunch.** Here's how this works. Act like you're going to get out of bed by engaging your abs and lifting your head and shoulders off of the bed. Immediately change your mind and lie back down. Repeat 10 times.
- **Sexercise!** Getting it on with your partner can be a workout as long as you're willing to rip off your lazy pants and exert a little energy. A recent study found that, on average, sexual activity burned four calories per minute for men and three per minute for women. Twenty-five minutes in the sack can add up, but a quick romp won't exactly cut it, and lying there lifeless definitely doesn't count.

Sure, it's nice to veg out at the end of a long day, long week, or long five minutes. But the more you move the better you'll feel in mind, body, and spirit. So start small with the even easier exercises above. Pretty soon you might be surprised to discover that you actually feel motivated!

How to Apply This Information

To begin incorporating more fitness into your life:

1. Start by reviewing your vision statement and SWOT analysis for clues about which factors or circumstances are interfering with your ability to reach your fitness goals.

2. Focus on the one or two areas that are most impacting your nutrition. For Carol, the factors most interfering with her ability to get fit are her limited budget and busy schedule.

3. Based on what you learned in this chapter, identify your strategy for incorporating more fitness into your life and create your action plan. See some sample actions steps below.

Sample Action Steps Carol Might Take:
- Set an alarm 30 minutes earlier to make time for exercise in the morning.
- Ask Susan from the office if she wants to power walk during lunch.
- Purchase a new fitness DVD or check one out from the library.
- Get a pedometer.

Other Sample Action Steps to Incorporate More Fitness Into Your Life:
- Take Jill's Fitness Personality Quiz.
- Sign up for a gym membership.
- Schedule a free consultation with a personal trainer.
- Sign up for a 5K run.
- Download a fitness app to track exercise goals.
- Find a fitness buddy.
- Sign up for an introductory strength training class at the gym.
- Purchase a new pair of sneakers.
- Buy a piece of home cardio equipment, such as an elliptical, treadmill, or bike.

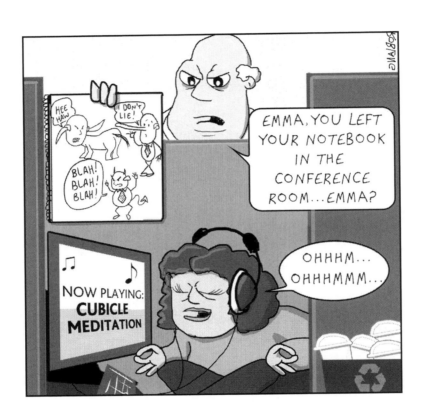

CHAPTER 13

Pink Slip Your Worries: Stress Management and Self-Care

Businesses know what it's like to deal with stress.

Every day they face increased competition, market volatility, and the growing scrutiny of social media. This all filters down to individual employees, who, in addition to the above stressors, are also dealing with longer hours, job insecurity, and—thanks to the invasiveness of mobile technology—the expectation to be "on call" virtually 24 hours a day.

Savvy companies know that true success depends on the well-being of their employees. Employee stress leads to reduced productivity, increased turnover, greater levels of absenteeism, and higher health care costs—all of which add up to create the biggest business stressor of all—a massive cluster of growing financial uncertainty.

That's why more businesses are taking notice and introducing perks to help employees unwind and chill. To help foster better work-life balance, some companies are offering catered meals, Fido-friendly environments, nap rooms, weekly massages, fitness facilities, increased time off, and flexible telecommuting options, among other creative solutions.

Just as the business world is being proactive in offering stress management programs on the job, individuals need to do the same thing for themselves. It doesn't matter whether you are in the home, out of the home, or at home—when you work yourself into the ground and push your brain and body to the brink, you pay a price.

Just Ask Peter (Again)

By now you should be familiar with Peter. You might recall that his goals centered around having more energy, and one of the biggest reasons he was feeling so drained was due to work-related anxiety and looming deadlines interfering with his sleep. When Peter formulated his vision and performed his SWOT analysis, he identified that work stress was the cause of his chronic sleep interruptions.

Now go back and look at your vision and SWOT analysis. Do you see any ways in which stress could be impacting your wellness?

Types of Stress

Stress comes in many forms and not all of it's bad. It keeps you alert and helps you strive to reach new goals. In that way, stress is an important and meaningful part of life. At some point, though, when it feels like you're drinking from a fire hose, stress stops being helpful and starts becoming a nuisance, damaging your health, your mood, your productivity, your relationships, and your quality of life.

In Chapter 9, I briefly outlined the three major types of stress that tend not to be so helpful, including:

- **Chemical stress.** This encompasses nutritional stress as your body tries to digest, assimilate and metabolize the crap you eat, drink and smoke. It also includes exposure to pesticides, pollution and other environmental toxins found in our air, water and food supply.
- **Mental stress.** Usually this form of stress results from our reaction to external influences, such as relationship or family issues, financial uncertainty, work stress, and during other times of loss, transition, or lifestyle change. Even positive major life changes can be super stressful, such as getting married, being pregnant, having a baby, or raising kids—whether they be threenagers or teenagers.

- **Physical stress.** This includes any form of bodily inflammation, structural problems, chronic pain, or sickness. Sources of physical stress tend to be internal and can occur when someone hasn't gotten enough sleep, doesn't exercise enough, exercises too much, or experiences an injury.

What Happens When You Are Stressed?

Stress is a physical response to threatening events or circumstances that upset you in some way. When you sense danger—whether real or perceived—your body's natural fight-or-flight mechanism kicks in to protect you, pumping out the stress hormones cortisol and adrenaline.

This response can save your butt in real-life emergencies. It's what gives you extra strength to defend yourself from a mugger and quickens your reflexes so you can slam on the brakes to avoid hitting a texting pedestrian with lightning speed.

The stress response also helps you rise to the occasion. Stress is what keeps you on your toes when giving a presentation, sharpens your attention during match point in your tennis game, or propels you to hunker down and meet that deadline when you'd rather be watching YouTube videos of cats pranking people who just had their wisdom teeth removed.

But today, with too many balls in the air at any one given time, many of us are experiencing a state of chronic stress. All the strain is hard on the body and mind and affects everything from your blood pressure to your digestive tract and your immune system.

Common symptoms of stress include fast, shallow breathing, sleep disturbances, excess sweating, stomachaches, nervous twitches (such as the infamous eye twitch!), teeth grinding, fatigue, food cravings, and more. All these reactions to stress sap our energy, leaving us feeling depleted, lethargic, and often irritable.

Extreme stress can lead to other even more dangerous repercussions, such as inflammation, weight gain, painful digestive issues, and even disease.

You've probably noticed in your own life that the more stressed you are, the more susceptible your body is to sickness. Nobody is immune. Since starting this book, while raising three kids and working as a health coach, I've been sick more times than I have in the past several years put together. That's no coincidence!

When you run out of bandwidth to cope with everything that's coming at you, your body will let you know one way or another. The question is—do you stop long enough to listen to it?

Knowing Where to Start

It's not about ridding stress from your life. To some degree, stress is necessary. But it's important to develop tools around managing stress so that you can stay in control of your mental, physical, and emotional well-being as often as possible.

Let's turn back to Peter. To get a handle on those sleep interruptions, he needs to reduce his stress. If he creates some action steps around lowering his work-related mental stress, he should be able to begin sleeping more soundly.

Top Strategies for Managing Stress

There are four strategies you want to focus on when trying to manage your stress:

1. **Identify your triggers.** The first step to managing stress is to figure out what's causing it in the first place. Trigger events might include the kids not getting ready for school on time, a hectic work travel schedule, a tense relationship with a family member, an annoying co-worker, concerns over being house poor, incessant sibling squabbles, or a tween who insists on acting like an alien, to name a few options.

   - *Start a stress journal.* One effective and easy way to hone in on your specific stress triggers is to start a stress journal. This can help you keep track of the regular stressors in your life and your reaction to them. Each time you feel stressed, write it down in your journal. After a week or two, you will start to notice patterns and common themes. Record the following:

1. The time of the event
2. The trigger event
3. The level of stress you felt—on a scale of 1 to 10—with 1 being the lowest and 10 being the highest
4. How you felt, both physically and emotionally
5. Your coping response to the stress

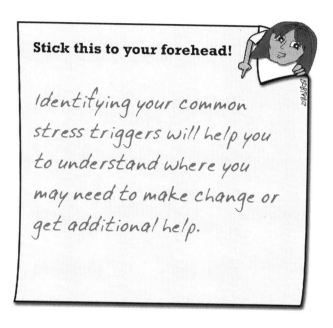

Stick this to your forehead!

Identifying your common stress triggers will help you to understand where you may need to make change or get additional help.

Here's a sample of what Peter's stress journal might look like. You can download a blank copy of this template at **jillginsberg.com/templates.**

PETER'S STRESS JOURNAL

When Peter analyzes his journal to identify common triggers, he will easily be able to see that work was the cause of his stress at least three out of five times.

Time	Trigger event	Level	Symptoms/ reaction	Coping response
7:30 a.m.	I locked myself out of my car.	8	Quick heartbeat. Sweating.	Kicked the car, then called a locksmith.
9 a.m.	I was late for the quarterly meeting with the CEO.	8	Shortness of breath. Anxious about impact on my career.	Talked with my friend about it and felt better.
3 p.m.	The deadline for a big client report is looming.	7	Headache. Lost my temper with my assistant.	Went outside to get some fresh air. Then stopped at the vend-ing machine for some chocolate.
8 p.m.	My boss called to check on the sta-tus of the report.	8	Shortness of breath. Headache again. Tension in shoulders.	Drank a beer.
2 a.m.	Neighbors are having a loud party.	7	Angry. Frustrated.	Tossed and turned. Then yelled "shithead!" out the window. Twice.

Once you review your journal you might notice that your stress is being triggered most often by your kids, your spouse, your job, concerns about money, or by another source.

2. **Avoid the source of unnecessary stress.** Not all sources of stress can be avoided (you can't give your kids away or start printing money at home!) but you might be amazed at how much can be dodged if you put your mind to it.

   - *Skip out on draining conversations.* Negative people are every-where. They're at work, in the car pool line and probably even in your book club. Do your best to stay away from these energy vampires. Or stick your fingers in your ears and go "La, la, la, la, la." That works, too.
   - *Give people who stress you out a pink slip.* If someone consis-tently causes you to feel drained and stressed, try to figure out what you can do to make the relationship more fulfilling. If you

can't turn it around, limit the amount of time you spend with that person or kick them to the curb entirely. Not all relationships are meant to last a lifetime.

- **Take charge of your environment.** If evening news reports of road rage, shootings, genocide, poisoned water or missiles that were accidentally fired in our direction make you anxious, turn the damn TV off. If traffic's got you tense, take the scenic route or use Uber instead. If going to the grocery store gives you palpitations, do your food shopping online. Take full advantage of the many alternatives that are available to you.
- **Be your own executive assistant.** Use some of the tips you learned in Chapter 6 to manage your time more effectively. If you've got too much on your plate, move tasks that aren't truly necessary to the bottom of the list or eliminate them altogether. Delegate what you aren't good at, get help whenever possible with tasks that you don't enjoy, perfect the art of saying no so you can defend your time, set firm boundaries around your work hours, and demand that others respect your personal space.

3. **Change How You Respond to the Stressor.** If you can't dodge a stressful situation, try to alter your reaction to it. We may not have control over all stressors, but we do have complete control over how we perceive and react to them.

- **Look on the bright side.** Try to view stressful situations from a more positive place. Rather than raging about a traffic jam, look at it as an opportunity to enjoy some alone time, catch up with a friend on the phone or do some of those car exercises highlighted in Chapter 12. Or, instead of focusing on the fact that your deadline for making a big business proposal just got bumped up to this Friday, be thankful you just got your weekend back and make plans to go see a movie.
- **See the big picture.** Take stock of the stressful situation. Ask yourself how much it matters in the long run. Will you care a year or even a month from now that somebody left the coffee pot empty in the break room? Is the fact that your eight-year-old insists on wearing shorts to school in the dead of winter really worth getting upset over? If the answer is no, keep your perspective and don't allow yourself to get caught up in the moment.

- **Be assertive.** Instead of stewing over something, throw on your big-girl panties and deal with it head on. If someone's rubbing you the wrong way, explain to them how you are feeling and why. They'll probably appreciate your candor! Or if you've got only 10 minutes to walk your dog before you have to head to a meeting and you see your chatty neighbor heading your way, there's no need to get all anxious. Just say up front that you only have 5 minutes to talk or ask him to walk and talk at the same time. It's not rude. It's the truth!

- **Find a sounding board.** If something's got you worked up, reach out to friends, family, and peers and use them as a sounding board so they can help talk you down. If your overbearing mother-in-law buys a one-way ticket to visit you, a phone call to your best friend to vent can make all the difference. Not to mention she has a spare room!

4. **Invest in yourself.** Let's be real, this is easier for some people than others. If you have little kids you can't even pee without an audience. You barely have time to brush your teeth or your hair. So it's hard to imagine how you could possibly have time to fit in self-care. But whether you're a busy executive, a busy parent, or both, everyone can find a few free minutes to nurture themselves.

    - **Connect with yourself.** Whether it's a spiritual practice, an art project (I hear there's a sale on adult coloring books), or journaling, connect with the most important person in your life—you!—and tune into your inner desires and passions.

    - **Work it out.** Hit the gym. Go for a run. Do a few quick sets of push-ups. Breaking a sweat helps you blow off steam and gives you that post-workout endorphin rush—both of which reduce stress in a big way.

    - **Try a relaxation technique.** You don't have to dive head first into meditation. Start by doing some deep breathing whenever you feel yourself getting anxious or tense. Take 2 minutes and simply notice your breath going in and out to help center yourself and calm down. Or try biofeedback, hypnosis, or music therapy.

    - **Get enough zzz's.** I don't know about you, but I need a solid eight hours to keep my bitch-switch flipped to the Off position. Do what it takes to get enough rest even if it means sometimes pretending to be in a deep vegetative state whenever the toddler wakes up in the middle of the night or the fourteen-year-old dog vomits.

- **Find the funny in it.** A good laugh lifts you up and boosts your body's feel-good endorphins. Lighten up by tuning in to your favorite sitcom, reading the comics, or chatting with someone who has a hilariously inappropriate sense of humor. (I'll be waiting for your call.)

- **Do something you enjoy every day.** It might be getting outside for a morning walk, cuddling in bed with your kid or dog, or quietly reading by the fire. Whatever you enjoy, pause for a few free minutes each day for activities that restore your energy. If you regularly make time for fun, you'll be in a better place to handle life's stressors when they inevitably come.

Here is a list of self-care ideas for you to consider:

30 Self-Care Ideas

Practicing self-care nurtures you on the inside, and outside, while allowing you to find your inner om.

1. Take a class you've always wanted to take, like dancing, cooking, Italian for beginners, photography, or pottery.
2. Try a new fitness class or choose something that allows you to exercise your mind and body at the same time, such as yoga, tai chi, or qi gong.
3. Take a nap.
4. Soak in a hot tub or take a bubble bath.
5. Try acupuncture.
6. Window shop.
7. Read a good book.
8. Laugh.
9. Meditate.
10. Go out on a day trip by yourself.
11. Keep a gratitude journal.
12. Listen to your favorite songs.
13. Hang with your pet.
14. Have a cup of herbal tea.

15. Get out in nature.
16. Get a massage.
17. Use essential oils and learn about the benefits of various ones.
18. Practice visualization or guided imagery.
19. Watch the sun rise or set.
20. Go for a walk on the beach.
21. Book a pedicure or manicure or both.
22. Practice deep breathing.
23. Do stretching exercises.
24. Do some gardening.
25. See a play, movie, or concert.
26. Ride a bicycle.
27. Treat yourself at one of your favorite restaurants.
28. Color, draw, or paint.
29. Swim, float, or relax in a pool.
30. Imagine you're in your happy place. Then go there!

Apply the coping mechanisms from this chapter to your own life and use your journal to notice how, over time, your response to stress changes. Not only are these tips useful in allowing you to monitor day-to-day stress, they could save your life during particularly trying times of the year. Like during the next sequel of "Close Encounters With Your Extended Family," also known as the holidays.

Five Ways Deep Breathing Will Keep You from Killing Your Family During the Holidays

Tis the season to be jolly. Fa la la la la, la la la la. Or that's what they say, at least. But tis also the season to be a basket case and go all Lizzy Borden on your family.

As much as the holiday season is known for being festive and joyful, it's equally known for being stressful and miserable. Combine the shopping frenzy, the pushy crowds, the pressure of Pinterest perfectionism, Uncle David's annual lecture on the benefits of circumcision, the non-stop parties, ceaseless head-splitting Christmas music, and the fact that the kids are home on winter break for Two. Solid. Weeks... and you're pretty much guaranteed to blow your ugly sweater top.

Luckily there's an easy tool to help you keep it together. Breathing exercises are a simple and super-effective way to reduce stress and tap into that inner Zen.

Here's why it can help you keep your cool:

1. **It's immediate.** When stressed, your breathing is typically shallow and you don't use your full lung capacity. That's because your brain thinks your body has better things to do—like help you escape from the hungry lion that's hunting you down. It has no idea that the reason you're really freaking out is because you just discovered you misspelled your own child's name on this year's holiday card, which, unfortunately, already got mailed. Oops.

   While your sympathetic nervous system is working overtime stimulating the flight-or-fight response in your body, deep breathing counters that response by increasing the supply of oxygen to your brain, promoting a state of calmness. This triggers an immediate relaxation response in your body that allows your heart rate and blood pressure to decrease, your breathing to slow, your muscle tension to ease up... and your mind to embrace the fact that you now have one hell of a great story to tell your son. Or not.

2. **It's easy.** Anyone can master deep breathing within just moments. Start by sitting up straight enough to make your third-grade music teacher proud and then rest your hands on your stomach. Exhale fully through your mouth. Breathe in deeply through your nose and into your belly, letting your belly fill with air. Hold your breath for a few seconds and then exhale through your mouth. The time it takes to exhale should be about twice what it takes to inhale. A good rule of thumb is Dr. Andrew Weil's 4-7-8 Exercise. Take 4 seconds to inhale your breath, 7 seconds to hold it, and 8 seconds to exhale. Repeat several times until you feel yourself settle down or you're no longer envisioning shoving your spouse face first into the blazing hot oven.

3. **It's portable.** Deep breathing can be used anywhere. You can discretely practice the simpler techniques, such as the one outlined above, in public without anyone even noticing what you're doing.

This means your deep breathing can be applied on the fly while traveling, at work, or even at a restaurant. The key is it to use it whenever anything upsetting happens, *before* you react. So the next time your little one uses a Sharpie to scribble satanic messages all over your late great grandmother's treasured tea towels, bust out some deep breaths and you'll be able to banish your nasty Joan Crawford-y alter ego to the land of wire hangers.

4. **It's preventative.** If you know you're heading into a stressful situation, take a few minutes to get yourself in the right state of mind. It's amazing how just a little deep breathing can help you honor your harmonious intentions. You're far less likely to be bated by your brother's favorite holiday game of one-upmanship. And the more you practice it—deep breathing, not one-upmanship—the faster your body will be able to trigger the relaxation response and bring your body and mind back into a state of happy equilibrium. Activate fake smile now.

5. **It's priceless.** Sure, it would be great to sign up for that two-week silent mediation retreat or hit the yoga mat every day, but these relaxation techniques can often be pricey and time-consuming. Many stressed out people don't have the funds or the time. Deep breathing doesn't cost a dime and it might just save you from your next major meltdown. So you'll never have to think twice or consult your budget before using it to help keep your stress levels in check.

Remember to breathe deeply and often this holiday season. You'll hardly flinch when your sister-in-law says, "That dress looks really good on you. Is it designed especially for plus-sized women?"

Still, you might want to put a padlock on the toolshed and eighty-six the key. Just in case that axe tempts you more than that second slice of pie.

How To Apply This Information

To begin managing your stress more effectively:

1. Start by reviewing your vision statement and SWOT analysis for clues about which factors or circumstances are interfering with your ability to relax.

2. Focus on the one or two areas that are most impacting your stress. For Peter, work stress is interfering with his ability to relax and sleep.

3. Based on what you learned in this chapter, identify your strategy for incorporating more relaxation into your life and create your action plan.

Sample Action Steps Peter Might Take:
- Start keeping a stress journal.
- Delegate some work responsibilities to direct reports.
- Schedule a meeting to talk to the boss about setting boundaries around work hours.
- Practice deep breathing when having trouble sleeping.

Other Sample Action Steps to Incorporate Stress Management Into Your Life:
- Block out an hour each week for massage, acupuncture, or some other form of self-care that occurs out of the house.
- Sign up for a new class—something fun, not stressful.
- Start a gratitude journal.
- Don't check email after 7 p.m.
- Begin each morning with a cup of tea and a walk.
- Take a bath before bed each weeknight.
- Stop watching the news at dinner.
- Limit conversations with that whiny friend.

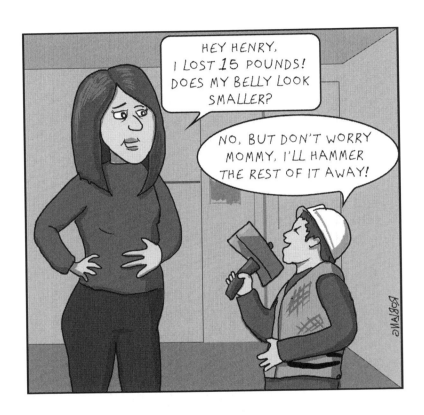

Your Future Wellions

Take a look around. Everywhere you turn, people are measuring success based on what's in their wine cellar, how well their stocks are performing, or the square footage of their walk-in closet (I mean—"dressing room").

You are among a growing cadre of enlightened people who now know better. Your yardstick for prosperity is different. Though you are responsible for a great deal, you understand that your most important job is to be self-healthy, happy, and fulfilled. Nothing is more valuable than that.

Now that you've completed this book, you are well on your way to reclaiming your health and feeling like a million bucks. You have devised concise goals and action steps to bring your wellthy vision to life. You understand how to avoid common pitfalls, and you're armed with sound wellness advice that you can immediately begin applying to your life.

Your Future Wellions—Final Thoughts
Don't stop once you've achieved your initial goals. Set your sights on even bigger ones. In the business world this quest to always do better is called "continuous improvement." It's what allows companies to ensure that their products and services keep pace with a constantly evolving environment.

Likewise, your needs will shift over time. To protect your future wellions:

- Conduct a self-assessment every six months to evaluate your progress and performance. Are you still following your Weekly Action Plan and keeping up with your Self-Healthy Living Schedule? Be honest about your triumphs and failures. Ask what you could be doing to better manage your wellions, and what your hopes are for the future. Then adjust your goals accordingly.
- Take a cue from the business world and make it a 360-degree assessment. Ask those in your immediate circle to weigh in on your progress. If you have children, make sure you ask them how your performance stacks up. Kids are like scales—they won't lie when you ask them if you lost weight. Or ask your dad, partner, best friend, or co-worker for feedback on how you are doing. (Don't bother asking mom. She will ooh and ahh over you no matter what. Lovely as this adulation may be, it's not particularly helpful when you are looking for unbiased reviews.)
- Speaking of family, friends, and co-workers—they will make becoming a Wellionaire more fun. Team up with them whenever possible. Embark on future goals together. The more the merrier!

Follow the roadmap you created in this book. It leads you directly to greater wellth. Though you may fall off track occasionally, take heart in knowing that you can always find your way again. Dust yourself off, get up off your ass(et), and refer back to your plan. Every now and then crack open this book again for a refresher.

Here's to your future wellions!

The Wellionaire's Glossary

80/20 Rule (n.) — a principle stating that one should commit to eating nutritious foods 80% of the time and allow themselves to loosen the reins the other 20% of the time.

Ass(et) (n.) — your buttocks.

Cup O' Laxative (n.) — super-duper, butt-explodingly strong coffee.

Energy loan (n.) — energy borrowed from another source, such as caffeine, sugar or other stimulants.

Fitness personality (n.) — your unique identity and preferences as it relates to fitness.

Flying by the seat of your yoga pants (v.) — winging it, while wearing comfortable clothes.

Good/Better/Best (n.) — a universal if slightly uninspired incremental system of improving something.

High-Five Rewards Roster (n.) — a list of bonuses to select from after you achieve a goal or milestone.

Jill's Magical Energy Scale (n.) — a basic 1 to 10 scale used to gauge an individual's energy level, with 1 being "I'm practically dead" and 10 being "I'm jumping off the walls and everyone around me wishes they were dead."

MBA-hole (adj.) — a graduate of Business School who displays annoying and contemptible qualities and often speaks in obnoxious business clichés.

Metric Matrix (n.) — grouped performance metrics that highlight areas of success as well as areas of weakness.

Mr. Lack of Direction (n.) — someone who wanders through life aimlessly with no clear sense of purpose.

Mr. Micro-Manager (n.) — someone who provides excessive and often unnecessary guidance or advice to subordinates.

Ms. Constant Critic (n.) — someone who has a habit of harshly judging, criticizing, or evaluating others.

No-Ninja (n.) — someone who is highly trained in the art of saying "No."

Nutritional stress (adj.) — the end result when a body has to digest, assimilate, and metabolize draining or nutrient-deficient foods.

Over-scheduler (n.) — someone who overfills their own schedule as well as the schedules of other innocents.

Pink slip (v.) — to dismiss, fire, or otherwise kick to the curb.

Self-health (n.) — the ability to foster better health for oneself.

Self-healthiest (adj.) — the maximum amount of self-health.

Self-Healthy Living Schedule (n.) — a weekly living tool that includes everyday activities and other important events essential to achieving health.

Six o'clock scramble (v.) — the shitastrophe that repeatedly plays itself out in homes across America, and elsewhere, when there is nothing planned for dinner.

Shitstorm (n.) — a chaotic situation.

Shitastrophe (n.) — a colossal catastrophe.

Stick This To Your Forehead (exp.) — a phrase meant to convey the importance of drilling an important concept or idea into your brain. Not to be taken literally.

Stress journal (n.) — a tool for recording stress triggers and other helpful notes.

Time thieves (n.) — people, places, or things that suck up your valuable time and resources.

Wellionaire (n.) — a person who is rich with energy, health, purpose, and joy.

Wellions (n.) — health and wellness-related riches.

Wellth (n.) — an abundance of energy, health, purpose, and joy.

Wellthcare (n.) — a more enlightened, holistic approach to healthcare in which the maintenance of the body and mind is more important than the accrual of wealth.

Wellth management (v.) — the act of managing one's wellth.

Wellth of Energy Equation (n.) — a mathematically-inspired expression for maximizing energy.

Glossary of Obnoxious Business Clichés

Back-burner (v.) — to deprioritize.

Balls in the air (exp.) — competing tasks being juggled.

Band-Aid solution (n.) — a temporary, inferior fix for a problem.

Bandwidth (n.) — the limits of your working capabilities.

Bang for the buck (n.) — value for the money.

Behind the eight ball (exp.) — at a disadvantage.

Bio break (n.) — bathroom break.

Boil the ocean (v.) — waste time on an endless task.

Carpool tunnel syndrome (n.) — the semi-vegetative state that occurs from sharing rides with people you don't want to be around.

Clock-suckers (n.) — an unproductive employee.

Ducks in a row (exp.) — organized things, items, or tasks.

Drinking from a firehose (v.) — taking on too much at once such that you become overwhelmed.

Eighty-six (v.) — discard or throw away.

Eleventh hour (exp.) — the last minute.

Fire drill (n.) — a perceived business emergency that usually isn't an emergency at all.

Head Honcho (n.) — the person in charge.

Low-hanging fruit (n.) — an easily achievable goal or target, or a problem that can be resolved with little effort.

Mouse potato (n.) — someone who sits in front of their computer most of the day and night.

No-brainer (n.) — something simple to understand or do because it requires little thought.

One-two knockout punch (n.) — two actions occurring simultaneously or very closely in time that result in successfully achieving a goal.

Outside the box (adj.) — creative or unique.

Phone it in (exp.) — to exert minimal effort.

Pie-in-the-sky (adj.) — idealistic but unlikely outcome.

PowerPointless (n.) — a type of presentation that is filled with nonsense.

Ramp up (v.) — to increase activity or exert more energy over a period of time.

Red flag (n.) — warning sign.

Ready! fire! aim! approach (exp.) — doing something prematurely.

Reinvent the wheel (v.) — to do something that's already been done before.

Road map (n.) — a plan.

Under promise, over deliver (exp.) — the act of purposely setting the bar low so that expectations can easily be exceeded.

Voluntold (v.) — when your boss or spouse assigns you an unpleasant task or project, often making it seem like the task or project was your idea.

Win-win (adj.) — a situation that is beneficial to all parties involved.

Glossary of Other Useful Business Terms

360-degree assessment (n.) — a system or process in which employees receive feedback from those they work closest with, typically including their manager, peers, and direct reports.

Accountability partner (n.) — a person who supports another person in keeping or achieving a commitment.

Alliance (n.) — a merging of efforts or interests between two or more parties.

Checks and balances (n.) — internal control mechanisms that guard against fraud and/or errors.

Chunking time (v.) — a process by which you focus on one task for a certain period of time in order to increase productivity.

Contingency plan (n.) — an alternate course of action that can be executed if a preferred plan fails or an existing situation changes.

Continuous improvement (n.) — an ongoing effort to enhance products, services, or processes.

Core competencies (n.) — a company's or enterprise's primary areas of focus or key strengths that distinguish it from its competitors.

Cost-benefit analysis (n.) — an analytical tool businesses use to assess the pros and cons of moving forward with an idea or proposal.

Economies of scale (n.) — the cost advantages enterprises obtain due to increased size, output, or scale of operation.

Hedging (v.) — the act of making a balancing or compensating transaction to protect yourself against making the wrong choice.

Inventory (n., v.) — a list of stock on hand, or making a list of stock on hand.

Joint venture (n.) — when two or more companies work together on a project or task but continue to maintain their separate identities.

Lean manufacturing (v.) — a philosophy that companies use to eliminate as much waste and excess cost as possible from the manufacturing process.

Limiting factor (n.) — a variable that restricts or limits production or sale of a given product.

Network (n.) — a group of people you affiliate with for professional or social purposes.

Outsource (v.) — delegate a task to an independent entity.

Performance review (n.) — a formal discussion about an employee's development and progress that typically occurs on an annual, semi-annual, or quarterly basis.

Plan B (n.) — a backup plan that can be implemented in case the original one (i.e., Plan A) proves impracticable or unsuccessful.

Point of diminishing returns (n.) — the point at which a benefit fails to increase proportionately with added investment, effort, or skill.

Productivity (n.) — a measure of output per unit of input.

Right-size (v.) — the act of reducing the work force to cut costs, become more efficient and increase profitability.

Risk management plan (n.) — a plan that identifies, assesses, and attempts to minimize risks.

ROI (n.) — abbreviation for return on investments.

SMART (n.) — a framework for setting goals that are Specific, Measurable, Achievable, Relevant, and Time-bound.

SWOT analysis (n.) — an acronym standing for Strengths, Weaknesses, Opportunities, and Threats that is often used by companies to better understand the environment in which they are pursuing goals.

Upgrade (v.) — to improve or enhance.

Variance analysis (n.) — a budgetary control tool that investigates the difference between actual and planned financial outcomes.

Vision statement (n.) — an aspirational description of what a business would like to achieve in the future.

Additional Resources

To download the templates in this book, and for additional resources, visit JillGinsberg.com/templates.

Visit JillGinsberg.com for more information on coaching and speaking engagements.

Interested in having Jill speak at your next event?

Jill is a natural born entertainer who motivates and inspires audiences with her fun, no-holds-barred style. Using personal anecdotes and lessons she's learned in her 15-plus-year career as a business woman and health coach, she keeps people laughing and on the edge of their seats—which only makes it easier for them to get off their ass(et) and reclaim their health.

She shares her compelling new system for implementing wellness change and her original brand of motivational humor during seminars and group workshops. Audiences include corporations, educational institutions, non-profits, writer and blogging conferences, and entrepreneurial groups.

For more information visit **JillGinsberg.com** or to book Jill at your next event please send an email to **bookings@JillGinsberg.com**.

Speaking Topics:

- Self-Health 101.whatever: 4 Simple Strategies to Stop Feeling Crappy and Start Feeling Radiant
- Finding Success Through Feeling Good: Lighthearted Stories and Lessons From People Who Have Done It
- Run Your Life Like a Boss: How Thinking Like a Manager Can Help You Take Charge of Your Health... And Everything Else
- You Are a SMARTy-Pants: How To Create Winning Wellness Goals So You Can Set Yourself Up for Success
- A Wellth of Energy: How to Leave the Land of the Living Dead and Wake Up to the Possibilities

- Get Off Your Ass(et): Four Simple Ways to Reclaim Your Health No Matter How Busy You Are
- Self-Made Wellionaire: Three Ways to Protect Your Ass(et)s So You Can Continue Feeling Like a Million Bucks

Group Workshop Series:

- Hedging Your Bets In the Kitchen: Meal Planning Principles Made Easy
- Get Wellthy The Fun Way: A Step-by-Step Guide to Getting Off Your Ass(et), Reclaiming Your Health and Feeling Like A Million Bucks
- A Wellth of Energy: How to Leave the Land of the Living Dead and Wake Up to the Possibilities—A Deeper Dive

Interested in coaching with Jill?

Want to work with Jill to accomplish your wellness goals? Interested in having her support your employees in thinking and feeling their best? For more support beyond the book, check out Jill's coaching options at **JillGinsberg.com/coaching.**

Interested in becoming a health coach?

This book was inspired by my experience at the Institute for Integrative Nutrition® (IIN) where I received my training in holistic wellness and health coaching. IIN offers a truly comprehensive Health Coach Training Program that invites students to deeply explore the things that are most nourishing to them. From the physical aspects of nutrition and eating wholesome foods that work best for each individual person, to the concept of Primary Food—the idea that everything in life including our spirituality, career, relationships, and fitness contribute to our inner and outer health—IIN helped me reach optimal health and balance. This inner journey unleashed the passion that compelled me to share what I've learned and inspire others.

Beyond personal health, IIN offers training in health coaching, as well as business and marketing training. Students who choose to pursue this field professionally complete the program equipped with the communication skills and branding knowledge they need to create a fulfilling career encouraging and supporting others to reach their own health goals.

From renowned wellness experts as visiting teachers to the convenience of their online learning platform, this school has changed my life and I believe it will do the same for you. I invite you to learn more about IIN and explore how the Health Coach Training Program can help you transform your life.

Learn more about my personal experience at **JillGinsberg.com/ resources**.

Acknowledgments

A huge debt of gratitude to my parents and siblings for your ceaseless love and weirdness. I thank my lucky stars every day that not a single one of you is normal. It makes me feel like I belong.

To my mother's womb, for providing nourishment and warmth, and for introducing me to my two best friends—my triplet sisters. Robyn, this book would be total shit without you. The attention you showed it, and me, is a wonderful gift that I will never be able to repay. Thank you for scrutinizing every single detail and for making it immeasurably better. You are the best sister money can't buy.

The biggest thanks goes to my family for your constant love and support, and for not taking it personally when I had to ignore you for days on end. Orly, your unwavering belief in everything I do, your positive attitude, and your ability to unintentionally misstate commonly used idioms and sayings amazes me every day.

Kids, I am eternally grateful to you for conditioning me to be able to work in any environment, no matter how insufferable or loud it may be. If not for the endless source of humorous inspiration you provide, I would have far less to write about.

Thanks to Jennifer Scharf for connecting me with my stellar editor, Amy Paradysz, who, in turn, connected me with the greatest thing to happen to this book—Flower of Life Press. Jane and Scott, thank you for believing in my book enough to publish it and for crafting an amazing platform in which to allow me and my wellthy vision to take flight. You are both my angels.

I can't forget The Institute of Integrative Nutrition, especially Joshua Rosenthal, for changing the way I—and the world—think about food. Lindsey Smith, thank you for skillfully guiding me and so many others toward putting our dreams on paper and for making anything seem possible.

To each of my clients, you have helped me to grow more than I could ever have helped you—technically, I helped most of you shrink. (Except those of you who chose not to listen to me—that's your own damn fault.) Thank you to Rob Lang for your sick sense of humor and hilarious illustrations, both of which make me feel like less of a freak. It takes one to know one.

Abby Lodmer, I can't help but think it was no accident that you were here the night I conceived the idea for this book. You are my muse. Wendy Thomson, you generously loaned me your home so I could hide from the world in order to meet my deadlines. (Now might be a good time to tell you that I had food poisoning while I was there.)

Special thanks to my book launch team and the ladies in my writing group for your sagacity and thoughtful commentary.

Finally, thanks to all the friends who took the time to inquire about my book, especially those of you who plan on buying *and* reading it. Your support means so much to me.[1]

---

[1] If you can't be bothered to buy the book and read it then you're probably a pretty terrible friend. But that's okay. We can still hang out together. As long as the drinks are on you.

About the Author

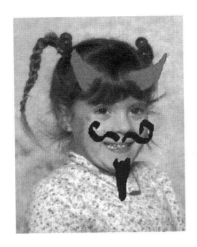

Jill Ginsberg is an author, speaker, health coach and mother of three wild little humans. After serving time in the trenches as a serial entrepreneur and former corporate manager, she combines her offbeat humor and business knowledge to teach busy people everywhere how to run their lives like a boss. Jill lives with her family in Seattle, Washington. Learn to get wellthy the fun way, and sign up for her newsletter at JillGinsberg.com.

About the Illustrator

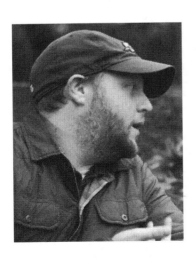

Rob Lang is a cartoonist and children's book author living with his beautiful wife and two zippy kids in Seattle. You can find his daily comic strip at UnderdoneComics.com.